Forza
THE SAMURAI
SWORD WORKOUT

Forza
THE SAMURAI
SWORD WORKOUT

KICK BUTT AND GET BUFF
WITH HIGH-INTENSITY SWORD FIGHTING MOVES

Ilaria Montagnani

Photographs by Bill Morris

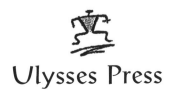

Ulysses Press

Published in the United States by
Ulysses Press
P.O. Box 3440
Berkeley, CA 94703
www.ulyssespress.com

ISBN 1-56975-478-0
Library of Congress Control Number 2005922405

Printed in Canada by Transcontinental Printing

10 9 8 7 6 5 4 3 2 1

Editorial/Production	Ashley Chase, Lily Chou, Claire Chun, Tamara Kowalski, Steven Zah Schwartz
Design	Robles-Aragón
Photography	Bill Morris
Models	Ilaria Montagnani, Irene Wong
Hair and Makeup	Roberto Gonzalez

Ilaria Montagnani is a Nike Fitness Athlete

Distributed by Publishers Group West

Please Note

This book has been written and published strictly for informational purposes, and in no
way should be used as a substitute for consultation with health care professionals. You
should not consider educational material herein to be the practice of medicine or to
replace consultation with a physician or other medical practitioner. The author and
publisher are providing you with information in this work so that you can have the
knowledge and can choose, at your own risk, to act on that knowledge. The author
and publisher also urge all readers to be aware of their health status and to consult
health care professionals before beginning any fitness program.

Table of Contents

part one

GETTING STARTED

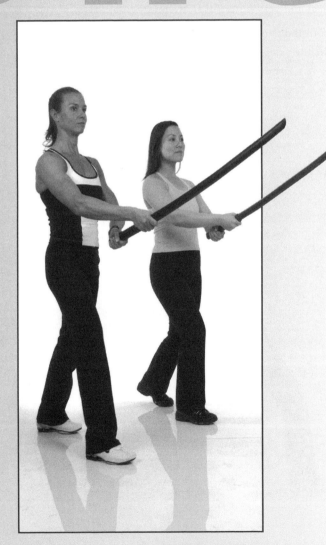

The Sword and the Warrior

There are many types of martial arts. I've studied several, drawn from traditions that originated in Japan, China and South America, but never has anything made me feel the way I did the first time I held a sword.

I've also trained in many sports and fitness disciplines, including swimming, rowing, running, weight lifting, diving and ballet. None of them compares to training with a sword.

It isn't that swordsmanship (or swordswomanship) is better than other martial arts, nor is it the ultimate fitness challenge. It's just that, as you will discover, there is something uniquely magical and very powerful in training with a sword.

Although both the philosophy and the practice of kendo, the "way of the sword," have their origins in the feudal Japanese military societies known as samurai, the method I

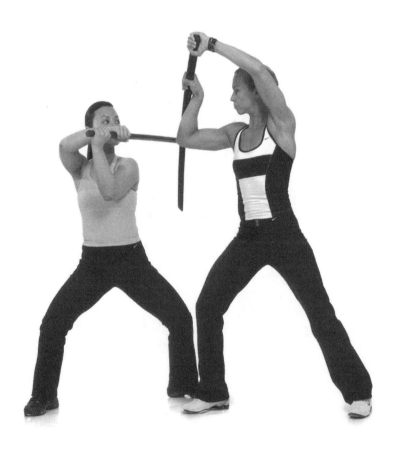

teach in my classes and in this book has nothing whatsoever to do with violence or bloodshed. Indeed, if your main purpose in studying martial arts is self-defense, you're better off studying kickboxing, because walking around on city streets armed with a samurai sword can get you in trouble.

Instead, sword training is all about integrating mind, body and spirit. It is mentally intense, physically tasking and, ultimately, spiritually rewarding. Through this practice, you will develop great strength and stamina as you learn a whole new dimension of speed and precision. A sword will teach you how to focus, to concentrate and at the same time to let go, to be in the present moment.

A sword will also teach you to have no fear. To be successful with a sword, you must find in yourself the desire to overcome fear. You will learn how to push past your limits, to be fully committed to your actions, and to find the determination in yourself to strive for more.

It is said that to be a successful swordfighter you must be calm, without fear, ready inside your heart and accepting, so that your actions can be natural and effortless. This means you must also learn not to try too hard, or you will never get there. Skill with a sword comes from the inside as well as the outside. Physical training alone won't do it. The mind alone won't do it. Both must work together. They unite in the sword, an instrument that represents both the journey and the destination.

The journey is a long one. I have chosen to take this journey with my sword and show many others the way. I want to show them—and you—how to push themselves, measure themselves, believe in and commit to what they want, find the determination, erase fear and ultimately achieve their dreams.

ABOUT THE INSTRUCTOR

Okay, by now you may be thinking that I sound like Yoda in *The Empire Strikes Back*—full of martial arts philosophy. But does it work in the real world? Let me start by telling you a little about myself.

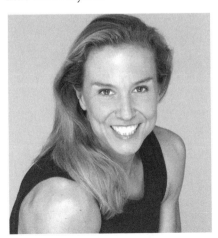

I began studying and practicing martial arts almost fourteen years ago. After getting my black belt in Karate, I became interested in the study of the sword, Japanese style. I devoted a lot of time to learning Aikijujitsu and Iaido, traditional Japanese swordfighting disciplines.

In 1995 I founded Powerstrike Inc., a fitness company designed to bring the essence of martial arts to fitness professionals and exercise enthusiasts across the world through unique workouts and training systems. Soon after, I harnessed the techniques I had mastered to create a modern sword fitness course which I have called Forza ("strength" in Italian, my native language). Drawing on samurai tradition, I teach a series of authentic sword sequences and movements including all the basic cuts and strikes.

Forza has begun to gain recognition as a powerful and unique form of training. I have traveled to many countries to teach it to instructors and fitness enthusiasts. Forza has given me the opportunity to meet people in Canada, Mexico, Sweden, Russia, Italy, Spain, Germany, Brazil and even Japan. Yes, that's right—Japan, where the Way of the Sword got its start so many centuries ago.

A LITTLE HISTORY

The samurai were a fearless, powerful force of warriors who ruled Japan for six centuries. The word samurai originally meant "to serve" and was first used to describe the personal servants of wealthy landowners in feudal Japan. As the central government of the country weakened, many of the landowners became warlords, protecting their subjects by the force of the sword. Thus, in the 12th century, the warrior class of samurai was born. Although the samurai and their masters faded away with the industrialization of Japan in the 19th century, their code of honor and their swordsmanship remain the source of the greatest Japanese legends, living on in the national spirit.

Although most samurai were men, women were also trained in the martial arts. The favored weapon for women warriors was the naginata, a swordlike weapon made of wood with a steel blade on the end, which was used in similar fashion to a sword but weighed less. Japanese legends tell of a number of female samurai warriors whose sense of honor and fighting spirit matched those of any man. Among the women samurai remembered in Japanese legend are Tomoe Gozen, wife of the famous samurai leader Minamoto Yoshinaka, and Hojo Masako, known as "the general in a nun's habit." Through most of the samurai era, Japanese women enjoyed more rights than women in most other cultures, including an equal right of inheritance.

In later periods, women warriors arose in time of need. For instance, in 1868, during the fighting between supporters of the Japanese shogunate and samurai loyal to the

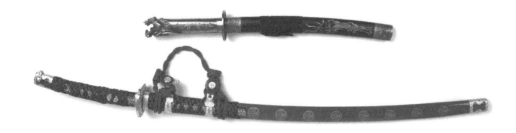

emperor (the era depicted in the recent film *The Last Samurai*), a group of 20 armed women stood up against an army of 20,000 men laying siege to Wakamatsu Castle. A monument to their leader, Nakano Takeko, stands in the Hokai temple in Aizu Bangemachi, Fukishima province. In 1877, the women of Kagoshima also rose up to fight against the imperial army when the male warriors were hopelessly outnumbered.

Today, though women train and fight as warriors in the United States and several other armies around the world, the sword has become obsolete as a weapon of combat. Yet the mystique of the sword lives on as a symbol of power, discipline and skill. It is these qualities, rather than violence, that form the basis of Forza.

THE LIVING SWORD

The sword was the samurai's most treasured possession. It was part of him. Swords were awarded by the Shoguns like medals for bravery, and legends even tell of samurai sacrificing their lives in battle to recover particularly powerful swords for their masters.

According to Japanese legend, the Sun Goddess, Amaterasu Onikami, gave the first sword to her grandson, Ninigi-no Mikoto, when she sent him down to rule the earth, and for that reason swords were the strength of Japanese rulers and their samurai until very recent times. Each sword was believed to have a life of its own, and the finest were thought to have mystical powers. Elaborate rituals developed for both the making and the handling of swords. Even today, there are companies in Japan that still make samurai swords, and the sword-smiths still use the same ancient techniques and rituals that their counterparts used in feudal times. These swords are not usually used as weapons, but are seen by collectors as objects of veneration representing an ancient and honorable heritage.

The sword was the samurai's most treasured possession.

For martial arts training, we do not use real swords, which can be enormously expensive as well as hazardous. To begin with, you can practice the exercises and routines in this book with any wooden stick about three feet long. A broomstick will do, but a little thicker stick would be even better. Paint the handle or wrap it with tape if you wish. Your stick does not need a tang ("hilt") because you will not be bringing it into physical contact with another body or sword.

A step up from the make-it-yourself stick are the wooden workout swords called bokken, which are available at any martial arts store or mail-order or internet supplier. These are typically made of hardwood and usually slightly curved like a genuine sword. Prices start at around $8.

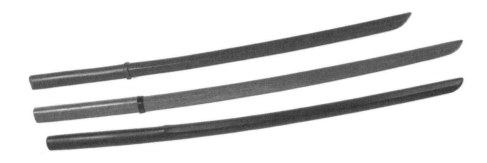

Even though you will not be using a steel sword in the practice of Forza, to obtain maximum benefit from this training it is best to accord your wooden "blade" the same respect that the samurai bestowed upon their swords.

PHYSICAL BENEFITS

The movements you will practice in a Forza session contain elements of both aerobic and anaerobic exercise. This is a very powerful combination. Aerobic ("with oxygen") exercise such as jogging, swimming or dancing burns calories from fat. However, it only continues to burn calories while you are exercising, and for it to have a continuing fitness effect you must increase either the speed or the duration of the exercise. Anaerobic ("without oxygen") exercise such as weight lifting burns calories mostly from carbohydrates, but as a side effect it increases your metabolic rate so that during periods of rest the fat burning process speeds up.

In Forza, the aerobic elements of the cuts and footwork operate together with the anaerobic elements of lifting and controlling the sword. To put it simply, it not only burns off fat while you are doing it; it also continues to burn fat after you've finished your

Forza utilizes every muscle in your body.

workout as you go about the rest of your day, making it an extremely efficient way of shedding unwanted pounds. A one-hour Forza workout will burn 300 to 500 calories.

Forza utilizes every muscle in your body. The moving of the sword, cutting and striking, and the leg workout of lunging and squatting bring the heart rate up in an intensive cardiovascular workout. At the same time, every time you strike, making the sword stop at the right height and target point makes for an isometric contraction of all upper body muscles. Controlling the force of the sword in motion acts as a powerful muscle building and shaping exercise.

MENTAL BENEFITS

Forza is a form of moving meditation. Controlling your sword requires a special kind of concentration that forces your mind and body to work together. Like other forms of meditation, it compels you to exist in the present moment, free from the distractions and mental chatter of everyday life, while developing your capacity for precision and deliberation. Get lost in the movement of each cut. Trying to perfect it, practicing it over and over, becomes a zone where we can get lost in deep concentration.

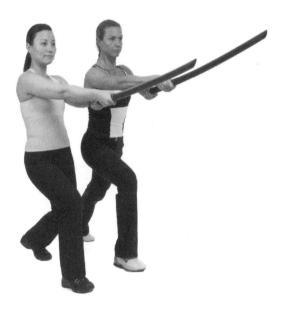

Like other forms of meditation, Forza not only enhances mental clarity but also helps us to eliminate unhealthy stress, restoring the body to a state known as "homeostasis" or balance. Medical science is only now beginning to realize that various forms of meditation, long practiced in Asia through martial arts and other methods, have profound physical effects. It helps us sleep and heal. It reduces high blood pressure and thus helps protect against heart attacks and strokes. It improves digestion and other glandular functions, including the sex drive. In fact, many holistic practitioners believe that most illness results from a state of physical imbalance, and that by restoring balance, meditation can help heal a wide variety of chronic conditions and activate the immune function. If you are skeptical about any of this, practicing Forza will quickly convince you of the fundamental oneness between your mind and your body.

Finally, Forza, like other forms of meditation, can act as a form of natural psychotherapy, providing an antidote for anxiety, panic and phobias. It has been proven that reducing levels of physical tension in the body makes people much less likely to suffer panic attacks and related symptoms. Many experts believe that meditation also slows the aging process, augmenting the effects of improved physical fitness. And of course, sword training imparts a wonderful feeling of self-confidence that further contributes to sound mental health.

No wonder the samurai always considered the way of the sword not as a destructive force but as a way of creating a better life.

SPIRITUAL BENEFITS

Spirituality is the most ephemeral of Forza's benefits, and also the most profound. In the samurai philosophy, the sword symbolized a tool for cutting down your own ego, cutting down your faults, fighting an internal battle with the aspects of yourself that are undesir-

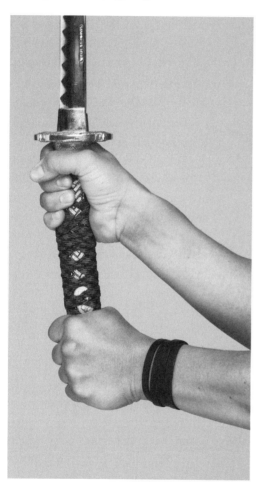

able, and making you more altruistic, caring, understanding of the world around you. The sword helps us become "higher," better human beings, fighting for the best in ourselves. Hours of practice and discipline, cut after cut, forge rightness within us just as they did for the ancient samurai men and women.

I was first attracted to the martial arts because I wanted to learn how to fight, to protect myself and my loved ones. Yet I learned over the years that through physical practice I actually steeled my own mind and spirit to better stand up to the challenges of life.

Being a martial artist is, to me, a way of life. Mind and body together develop a strong spirit that can overcome obstacles and has the determination to "fight" for more and better, whether it is studying better at school, being proud and efficient at your job, overcoming an addiction or laziness. In mysterious ways, the sword helps me smile and walk through everyday challenges without letting them pull me down, win me over, or take me away from loving life. Warriors are modest but unafraid. They do not shy away or hide from life's duties, and they extend their power far beyond the everyday routines of life.

We all have many battles. By that I do not mean that life is only war. I am not talking about bloodshed. I am talking about external confrontations, internal battles, struggles for self-improvement, all the dramatic incidents of everyday life. This all takes energy, a very strong will, determination and especially discipline. The practice of martial arts helps us to find the strength for this discipline.

That's why we have a saying, "In the dojos we train our spirit." It is the spirit of the warrior that I am talking about. The meaning and depth of learning how to fight on a ring or a mat goes far beyond a specific workout or match, beyond an individual opponent, beyond winning or losing. Our practice becomes a vehicle for us to become masters at facing conflicts.

The challenge is to create something better for ourselves. The victory lies in fulfilling our dreams. The place we fight our battles now is our everyday life.

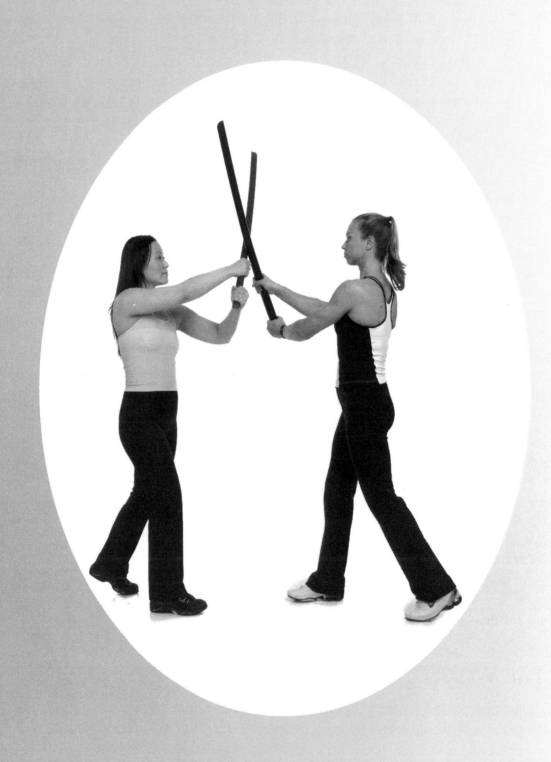

How to Use This Book

Once you have your bokken (this Japanese word means, literally, "wooden sword"), you need very little else to practice the exercises and routines in this book. Simplicity is one of the virtues of the Forza workout.

THE WORKOUT AREA

Forza was developed for practice in gyms and fitness facilities, which have a large space with no furniture or other obstructions but do not usually have particularly high ceilings. While a lawn or other outdoor practice space is ideal—you can practice with the sword and work on your suntan at the same time—it's not necessary. An empty basement room or an unfurnished spare bedroom can work just as well. If you're doing the cuts correctly, your sword should not hit the ceiling even when doing a full cut with the sword raised over your head. You can even do it in the living room if you move the furniture out of the way and make sure there's no danger of accidentally striking that prized antique vase or the dog. In short, any space that's large enough for uninhibited dancing is also adequate for practicing Forza.

In my Forza classes, I always use music. You can do the same at home if you wish; for some people practicing on their own, music provides energy and motivation; for others it may be distracting. In class I use "trance" music, which is strong but somewhat dreamy, helping students get lost in the motion.

WHAT TO WEAR

Any clothing that you would wear for other kinds of fitness workouts is perfect. What you choose to wear is not important as long as the clothing does not restrict your movements. However I prefer to wear something I like and feel comfortable in when I practice with the sword; it helps me get in the mood and focus at the same time.

As for shoes, you don't need to invest in fancy running shoes unless you already have them. Forza is a low-impact workout. Any footwear that doesn't slip when you lunge is just fine. You can even do this workout barefoot. However, stocking feet or high heels are not recommended.

THE WORKOUT PLAN

As with most workout plans, you can do Forza sessions daily, every other day or three days a week. Of course, the more frequent your workouts, the faster you will progress. If

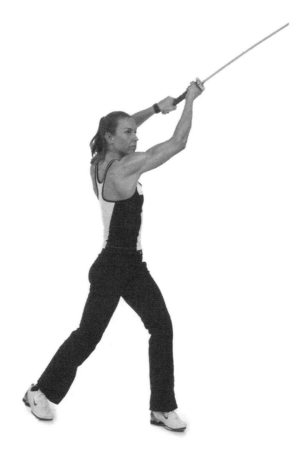

you're doing Forza as part of a weight-loss plan, daily sessions are best for speeding up your metabolism and burning calories. Start by working out 20 minutes, then progress to 30, then to 45, and if and when you can, push for an hour. Remember though that a little is always better than nothing—even if a little is only 10 to 15 minutes, that might just calm and free your mind.

Always start by warming up. After that, the first segment of this workout, "Basic Exercises," is to be done in the same sequence, with the same number of repetitions, every time you do them. Although this may sound kind of boring, you'll be amazed at how your precision and speed keep getting better and better. As you progress to the point where you can do the basic exercises smoothly and without thinking about them, move on to the "Advanced Exercises."

There are eight Advanced Exercises to choose from. Depending on how long you wish to work out, choose to practice one or two (or three at the most) per session. I always choose two Advanced Exercises for my hour-long workout classes, and have students repeat the exercises for 3 to 5 minutes straight at times.

The final segment of the workout, which I call "Routines," is the creative part. Each one is a series of choreographed moves—"choreographed" in the same sense that fight scenes in action motion pictures are choreographed move by move. Each one is more complex than the one before. Start with Routine #1 and practice it day after day until you can do it smoothly, without thinking. Then move on to Routine #2. (You can still go back and practice #1 in the same session if you wish.) When you have mastered Routine #2, move on to Routine #3 and so on. To learn a routine, practice it many times. To enjoy it and get the greatest benefits out of it, practice it over and over without thinking: just your body doing, your arms cutting, your legs guiding your breathing, which is strong but steady, your mind still.

When you have become proficient at all the routines in this book, try combining them or even making up your own.

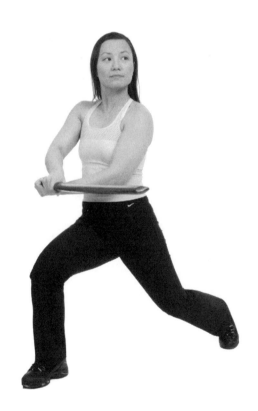

How to Hold the Sword

Before starting the actual workout it's important to become familiar with the sword. Think of it as a companion for your workout, not as a foreign object in your hands.

Hold the sword by placing your right hand all the way up with thumb and index just under the line that indicates the end of the blade and with left hand all the way down with left pinky by the rim at the end of handle. The blade should be turned away from you. Hands should never touch each other.

Wrists should be slightly turned in, as if starting to wring a towel, and always kept locked in that position. Try not to let the wrists turn outward as that will push the elbows out, loosen the grip on the sword and spoil the precision of the cut.

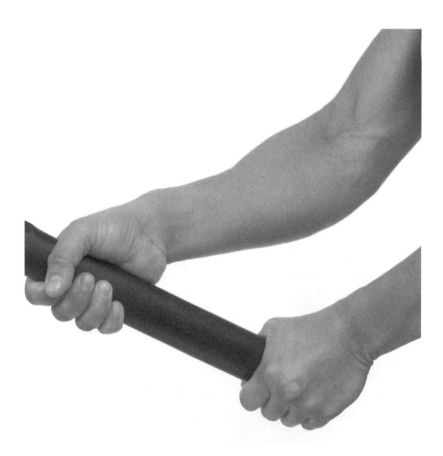

Both elbows should be bent and always remain bent in each cut—this is very important because when we let our elbows straighten out we lose the precision and the power of the cut as the force of the move gets transferred to the forearms and neck. Keeping the elbows bent makes us perform each move with our whole body, using the legs, back, chest, shoulders, arms and, of course, the abdominals.

THE MASTER HAND

In a regular sword class in a dojo or martial art hall, the master hand—the hand that holds the sword higher on the handle—will always be the right hand. For fitness purposes, in this book (as in all my classes) we will perform each cut, exercise and routine with the right hand on top first and then with the left hand on top to balance the workout and work both sides of the body evenly.

Always keep in mind that no matter which hand is on top, both arms as well as the shoulders and chest and back muscles should work evenly. The bottom hand should pull while the top hand pushes, and each muscle should contract strongly and evenly, stopping the sword at the proper point.

Exercises will be explained and illustrated only with the right hand as the master hand. To perform them with the left hand on top, just reverse the grip and repeat each cut and exercise as a mirror image of the right side.

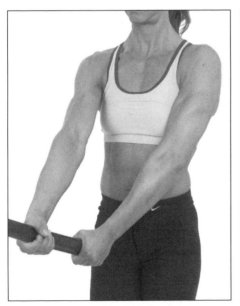

Incorrect Grip: Don't hold the sword like this, with straight arms.

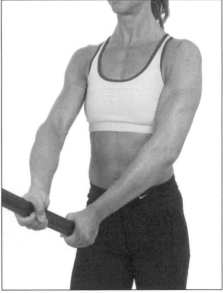

Correct Grip: Your elbows should be bent, like this.

On Guard

Each cut starts from the On Guard position: With the feet together or in any other position, the tip of the sword at eye level, the elbows slightly bent and the shoulder relaxed, aim at an imaginary opponent.

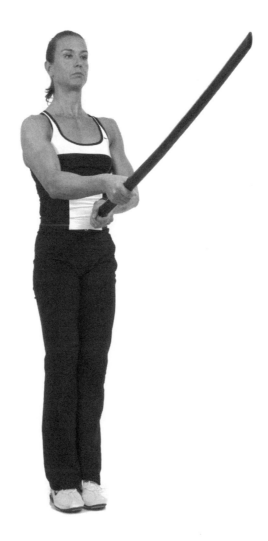

The On Guard position indicates the beginning of an attack. It shows that you are ready, not distracted or out of focus. It is considered disrespectful to take the On Guard position toward any person unless you intend to engage in a full fight.

Footwork

In this section I will explain and illustrate the various stances and leg positions. There are not many, so they are easy to remember.

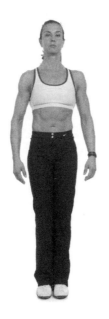

FEET TOGETHER STANCE: Your feet and legs are together, with knees slightly bent, abdominals contracted, and gluteus squeezed and tucked in.

RIGHT STANCE OR RIGHT STEP: Your right leg is in front, with your feet hip distance apart, like a regular step but with the knees slightly bent, left heel slightly up, abdominals contracted and gluteus squeezed and tucked in.

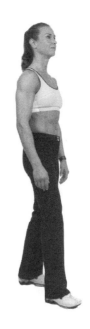

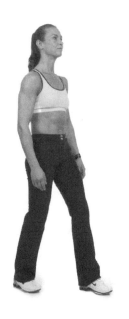

LEFT STANCE OR LEFT STEP: Your left leg is in front, with your feet hip distance apart, like a regular step but with the knees slightly bent, right heel slightly up, your abdominals contracted and your gluteus squeezed and tucked in.

SQUAT OR SAMURAI STANCE: Move into a squat position with your feet slightly turned out and wider than shoulder width apart. Your back should be straight, your abdominals contracted and your gluteus squeezed and tucked in.

RIGHT SQUAT: Sidestep right into a squat.

LEFT SQUAT: Sidestep left into a squat.

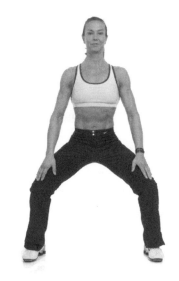

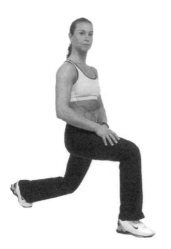

RIGHT LUNGE: Step forward with your right leg into a lunge with your feet shoulder width apart (not on a straight line). Your back should be straight, your abdominals contracted and your gluteus squeezed and tucked in.

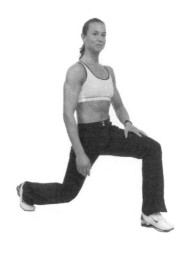

LEFT LUNGE: Step forward with your left leg into a lunge with your feet shoulder width apart (not on a straight line). Your back should be straight, your abdominals contracted and your gluteus squeezed and tucked in.

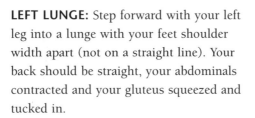

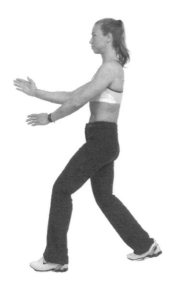

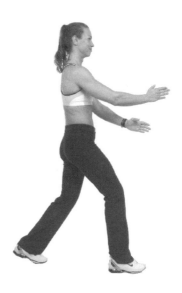

PIVOT: Keeping your feet in place, spin around 180° so that your back foot becomes your front foot, and vice versa.

part two

WARM-UPS & EXERCISES

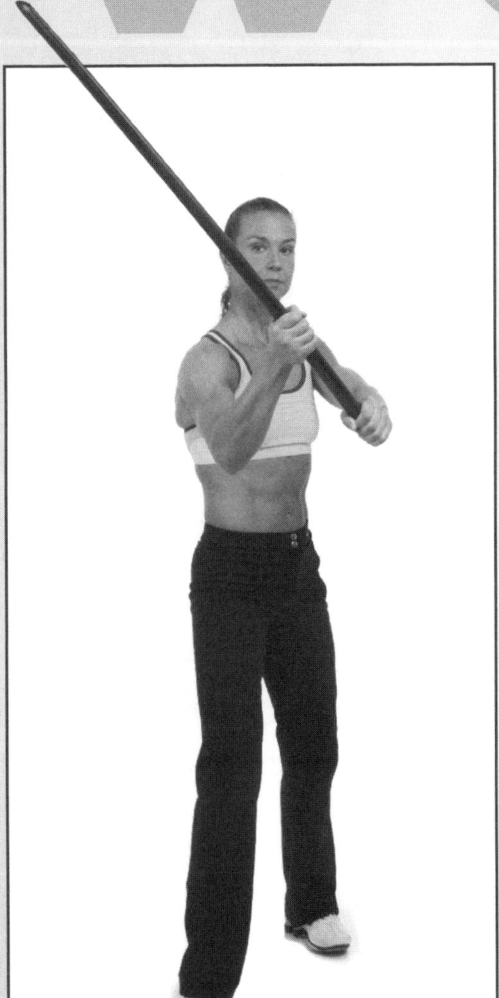

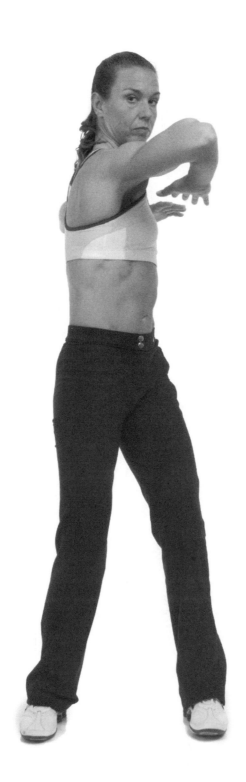

WARM-UPS

Each routine combines several of the exercises you
have practiced into a smooth sequence of choreographed movements. Practice the first routine
repeatedly until you can do it easily without looking
at the book. Then, proceeding at your own pace,
move on to the next routine. Later you may wish to
combine several routines into a longer one or
experiment with creating your own routines.

WARM-UPS

1

Rotate your ankles in both directions with the ball of the foot on the floor.

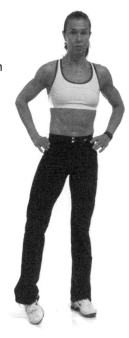
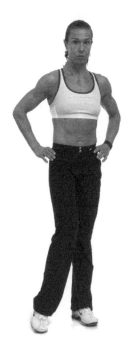

3

Rotate your hips in both directions.

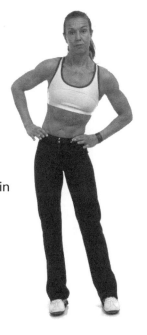
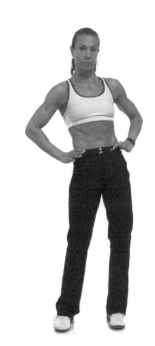

2

Rotate your knees in both directions with your hands just above them.

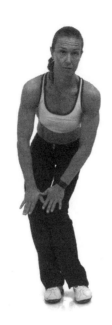

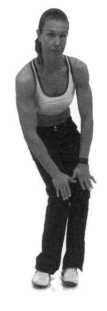

4

Rotate your upper body to warm up your waist and lower back.

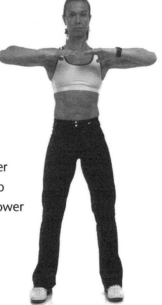

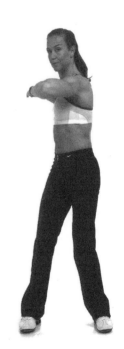

continued on next page ⟶

5

Slowly and separately rotate your right arm and then your left arm forward.

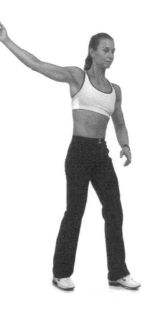
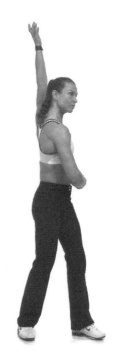

7

Stretch your wrists palm up, then palm down, and rotate a few times.

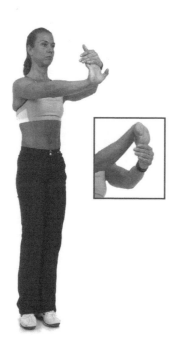
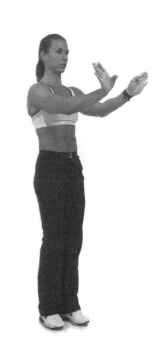

6

Look side-to-side to
warm up your neck.

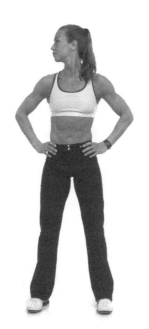
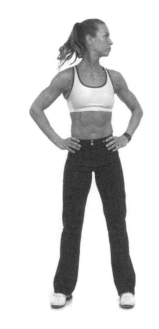

8

Roll your shoulders
back and front.

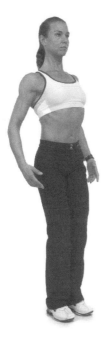
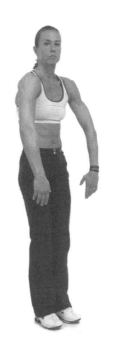

Now you're ready. . .

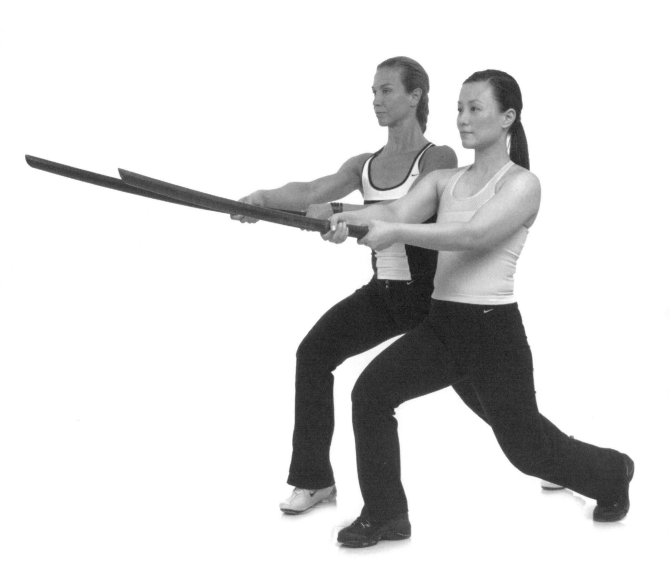

BASIC
EXERCISES

Pick up your sword and start the basic exercises.
Each move will warm you up even more and pre-
pare you for advanced exercises.

In the basic exercises, perform each cut between
three and five times using the right hand first as
master hand. (This means the right hand is on top.
See the section Holding the Sword.) Then repeat
with the left hand as master hand. Practice the
moves in a stationary position, without stepping
into the cut. Start slowly and strike lightly, as if cutting through clouds or cotton.

Basic Exercise #1:

HALF CUTS

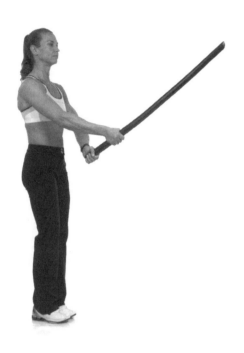

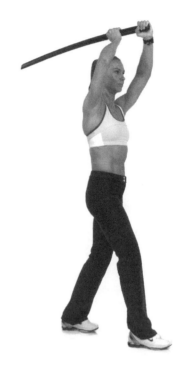

1. Start in the **On Guard** position with your right hand on top.

2. Take a **Right Step** forward and raise the sword high above your head and parallel to the floor. Your elbows should be bent and framing your face.

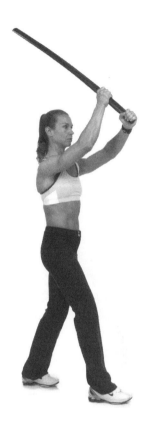

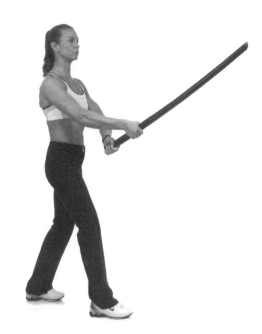

3. Visualize an imaginary line from the top of the head to neck level. Strike down following the center line of your body.

4. End the strike with the sword tip at throat height and the hands in front of the solar plexus, left hand close to the body and elbows bent.

Perform the exercise three to five times with your right hand on top. Then switch sides and repeat the exercise again with your left hand on top, substituting Left Step for Right Step, etc.

Basic Exercise #2:

FULL CUTS

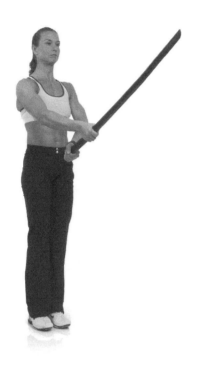

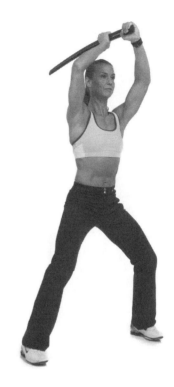

1. Start in the **On Guard** position with your right hand on top.

2. Sidestep **Left** into a **Squat** and raise the sword high above your head and parallel to the floor, elbows bent and framing your face.

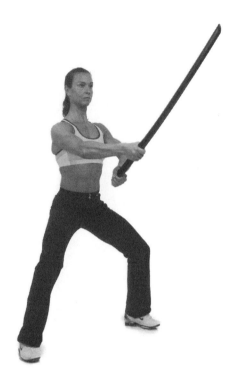

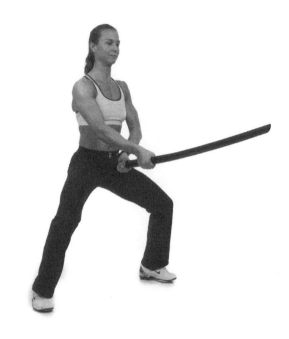

3. Visualize an imaginary line from the top of your head to your navel. Strike down following the center line of the body.

4. End the strike with the sword tip at navel height, hands in front of the belly, sword parallel to the floor, left hand close to the body and elbows bent.

Perform the exercise three to five times with your right hand on top. Then switch sides and repeat the exercise again with your left hand on top, substituting left for right.

Basic Exercise #3:

DIAGONAL 1 HIGH CUTS

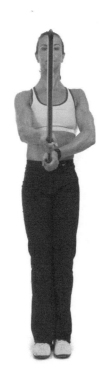

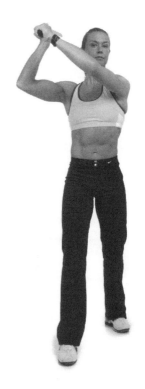

1. Start in the **On Guard** position with your right hand on top.

2. Take a **Right Step** forward and bring the sword up by the right side of your head, high above the temple, with the tip slightly higher than your hands and your eyes over your left forearm.

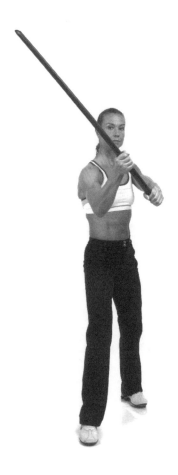

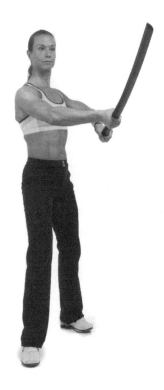

3. Visualize an imaginary line from right to left across the head, stopping in front of the left shoulder. Push from the right hip and shoulder. Lift your right heel and pull back from your left shoulder, striking with your elbows bent.

4. End the strike with the tip of the sword in front of your left shoulder, tip facing forward.

Perform the exercise three to five times with your right hand on top. Then switch sides and repeat the exercise again with your left hand on top, substituting Left Step for Right Step, etc.

Basic Exercise #4:
DIAGONAL 2 HIGH CUTS

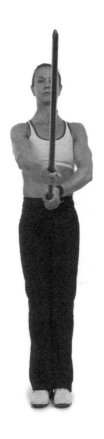

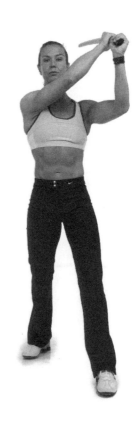

1. Start in the **On Guard** position with your right hand on top.

2. Take a **Right Step** forward and bring the sword up by the left side of the head, high above the temple, the tip slightly higher than your hands, and your eyes over your right forearm.

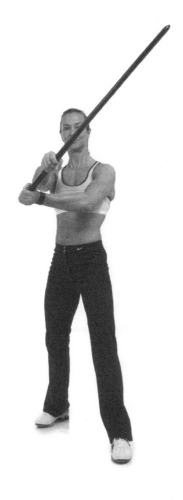

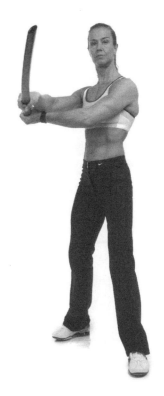

3. Visualize an imaginary line from left to right across th head, stopping in front of your right shoulder. Push from your left hip and shoulder, lift the left heel and pull back from your left shoulder, striking with the elbows bent.

4. End the strike with the tip of the sword in front of your right shoulder, tip facing forward.

Perform the exercise three to five times with your right hand on top. Then switch sides and repeat the exercise again with your left hand on top, substituting Left Step for Right Step, etc.

Basic Exercise #5:
DIAGONAL 1 LOW CUTS

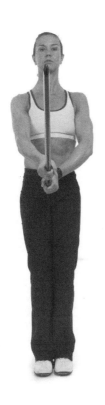

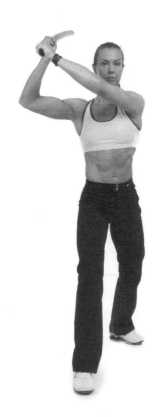

1. Start in the **On Guard** position with your right hand on top.

2. Take a **Right Step** forward and bring the sword up by the right side of the head, in line with the temple, with the tip behind and in line with the handle and your eyes over your left forearm.

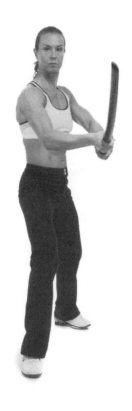 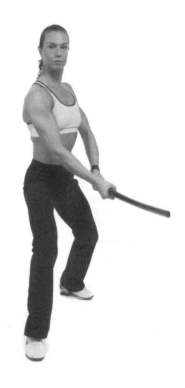

3. Visualize an imaginary line from right to left across the body. Push from your right hip and shoulder, lift your right heel, turning into a squat, and pull back from your left shoulder, striking with your elbows bent.

4. End the strike with the tip of the sword in front of your left hip, tip facing forward.

Perform the exercise three to five times with your right hand on top. Then switch sides and repeat the exercise again with your left hand on top, substituting Left Step for Right Step, etc.

Basic Exercise #6:

DIAGONAL 2 LOW CUTS

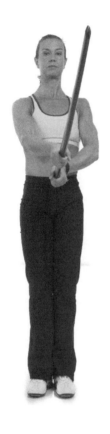

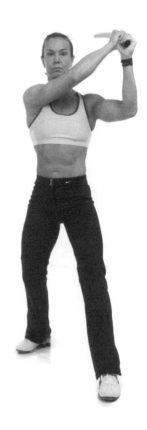

1. Start in the **On Guard** position with your right hand on top.

2. Take a **Left Step** forward and bring the sword up by the left side of the head, in line with the temple, with the tip behind and in line with the handle and your eyes over your right forearm.

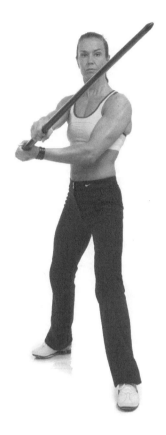

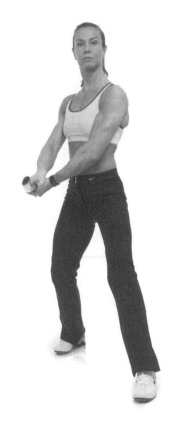

3. Visualize an imaginary line from left to right across the body. Push from your left hip and shoulder, lift your left heel, turning into a squat, and pull back from the right shoulder, striking with your elbows bent.

4. End the strike with the tip of your sword in front of your right hip, tip facing forward.

Perform the exercise three to five times with your right hand on top. Then switch sides and repeat the exercise again with your left hand on top, substituting Right Step for Left Step, etc.

Basic Exercise #7:

HORIZONTAL CUTS

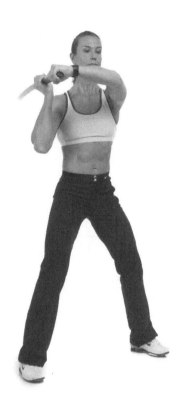 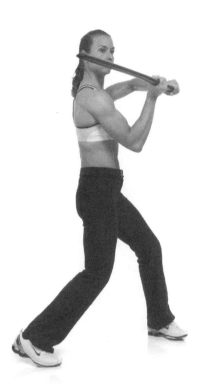

1. In a **Squat**, start with the sword tip behind your right shoulder and the handle in front of the right shoulder, holding the blade parallel to the floor.

2. Visualize an imaginary line across your shoulder at neck level. Rotate your right hip, lift your right heel and perform the cut, keeping the blade perfectly parallel to the floor.

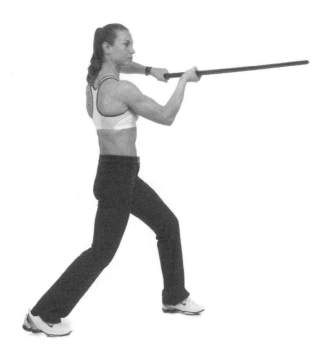

3. End the cut with the sword tip in front of your left shoulder, keeping your shoulders relaxed and your left elbow higher than your right elbow.

Perform the exercise three to five times with your right hand on top. Then switch sides and repeat the exercise again with your left hand on top, substituting left shoulder for right shoulder, etc.

Basic Exercise #8:
Reversed Horizontal Cuts

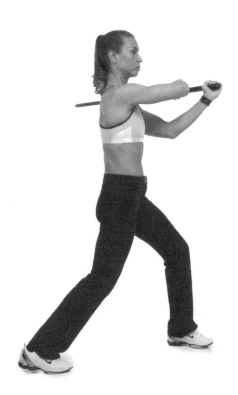 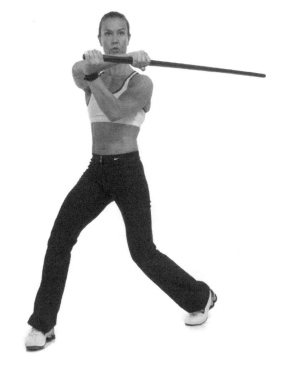

1. In a **Squat**, start with the sword tip behind your left shoulder and the handle in front of your left shoulder, blade parallel to the floor.

2. Visualize tracing a half circle around your shoulders, parallel to the floor. Rotate your left hip, lift your left heel and perform the cut, keeping the blade perfectly parallel to the floor.

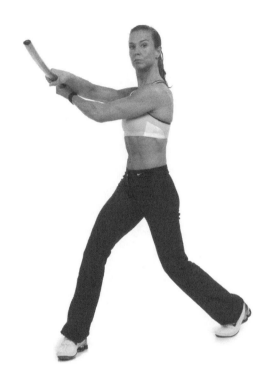

3.   End the cut with the sword tip in front of your right shoulder, keeping your shoulders relaxed and your right elbow higher than your left elbow.

Still in a Squat, perform the exercise three to five times with your right hand on top. Then switch sides and repeat the exercise again with your left hand on top, substituting right shoulder for left shoulder, etc.

Basic Exercise #9:

Low Horizontal Cuts

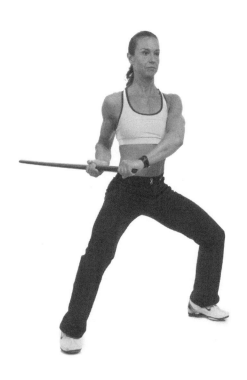

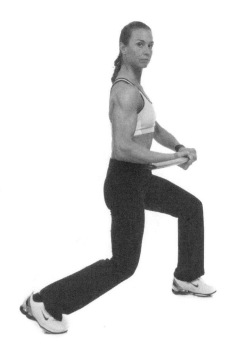

1. In a **Squat**, start with the sword tip behind the right side of your body at stomach level.

2. Visualize an imaginary line across the stomach with the blade parallel to the floor. Rotate your right hip, lift your right heel and perform the cut, keeping the blade perfectly parallel to the floor.

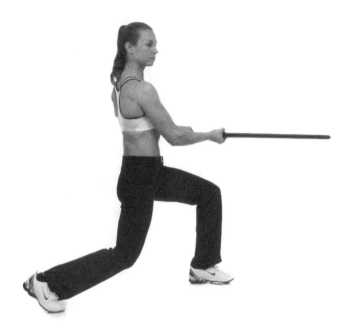

3. End the cut with the tip in front of the left side of your body, keeping your shoulders relaxed.

Still in a **Squat**, perform the exercise three to five times with your right hand on top. Then switch sides and repeat the exercise again with your left hand on top, substituting left hip for right hip, etc.

Basic Exercise #10:

Thrusts

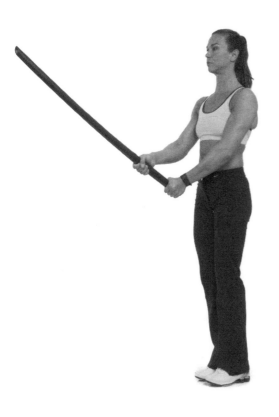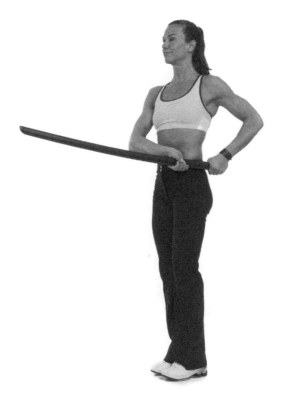

1. Start in the **On Guard** position with your right hand on top.

2. Bring your hands toward your left hip.

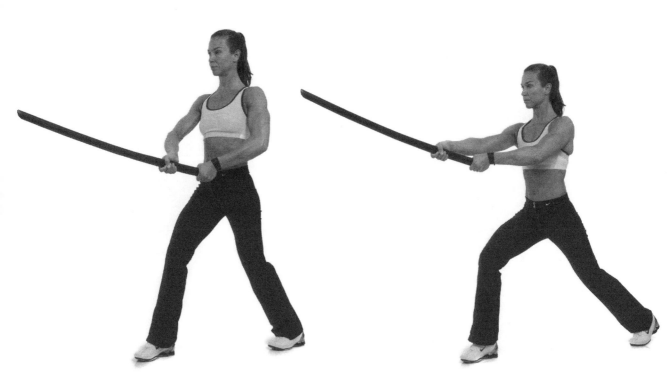

3. Strike by lunging with your right leg forward and pushing from your left hip and leg, thrusting the sword forward at neck level.

4. End with the sword tip at neck level and your elbows slightly bent.

Perform the exercise three to five times with your right hand on top. Then switch sides and repeat the exercise again with your left hand on top, substituting Left Step for Right Step, etc. You can also try performing the thrust at eye level or heart level.

Basic Exercise #11:

DIAGONAL 3 CUTS

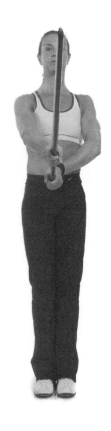
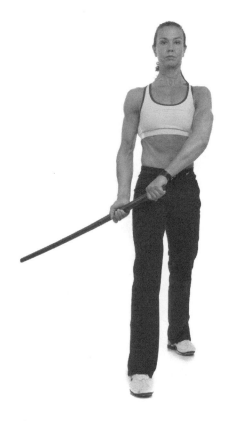

1. Start in the **On Guard** position with your right hand on top.

2. Take a **Right Step** forward and bring the sword down and behind your right leg.

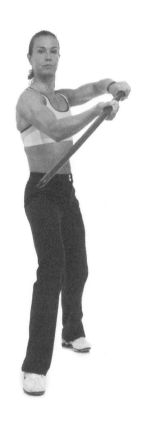

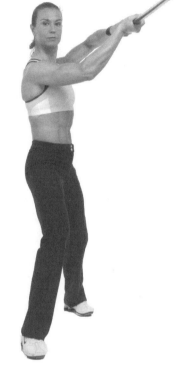

3. Visualize an imaginary line from your right hip up to your left shoulder diagonally across your body. Push from your right hip and shoulder, pull back from your left shoulder and rotate your body, striking with elbows bent.

4. End the strike with the tip of the sword in front of your left shoulder, tip facing forward, elbows bent with your left elbow higher than your right

Perform the exercise three to five times with your right hand on top. Then switch sides and perform the exercise again with your left hand on top, substituting Left Step for Right Step, etc.

Basic Exercise #12:

KENDO STRIKES

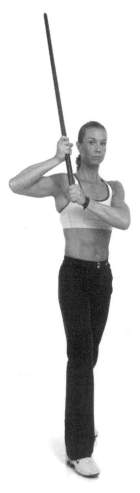 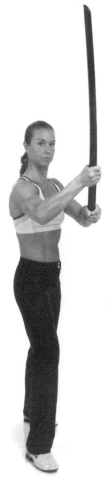

1. Take a right step forward and bring your sword behind your right temple, very high as if to strike a much taller opponent.

2. Strike out by slightly rotating your hips to the left, moving your arms quickly with your hands framing your face and your elbows bent.

Kendo is a Japanese word meaning "way of the sword." It is a traditional style of samurai swordfighting. In Forza, the term "kendo strikes" describes the shorter moves at either side of the head.

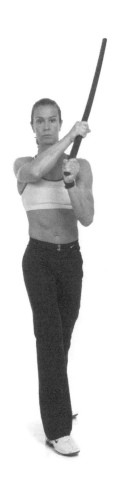

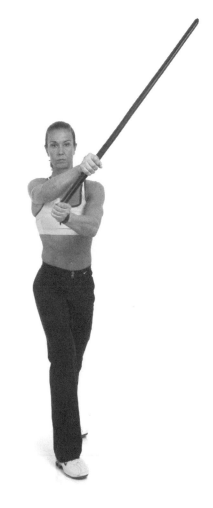

3. Bring your sword behind your left temple now.

4. Strike out again with elbows bent. Shuffle forward with each strike, keeping your right foot in front.

Perform the exercise for 30 seconds to a fast tempo with your right hand on top. Then switch sides and repeat the exercise again with your left hand on top, substituting Left Step for Right Step, etc.

Basic Exercise #13:

TWIRL WITH HALF CUT

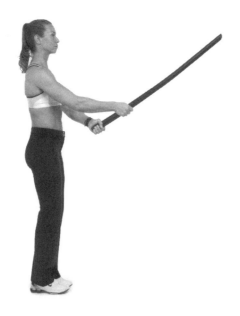

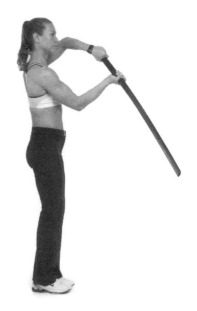

1. Start in the **On Guard** position with your right hand on top, **Feet Together**.

2. Drop your blade toward your right side, close to your body, with your fingers closed tightly.

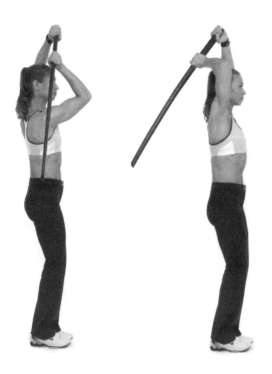

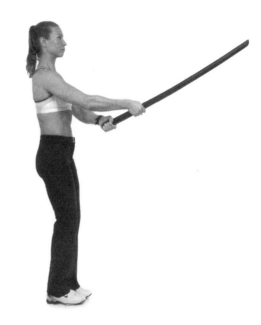

3. Twirl the sword over your right shoulder and behind your back, keeping your elbows high.

4. Strike a **Half Cut**.

Perform the exercise three to five times with your right hand on top. Then switch sides and repeat the exercise again with your left hand on top, substituting left side for right side, etc.

Basic Exercise #14:

TWIRL WITH FULL CUT

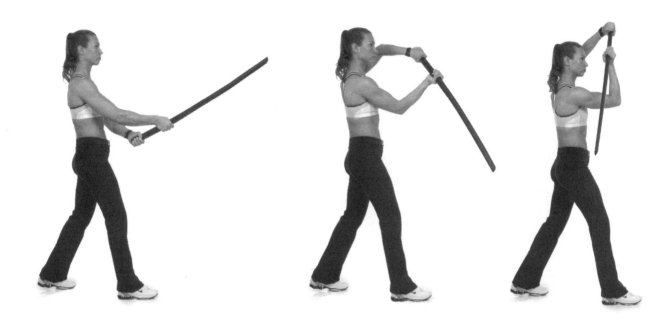

1. Starting in the **On Guard** position with your right hand on top, take a **Right Step** forward.

2. Drop your blade toward your right side, close to your body, with your fingers closed tightly.

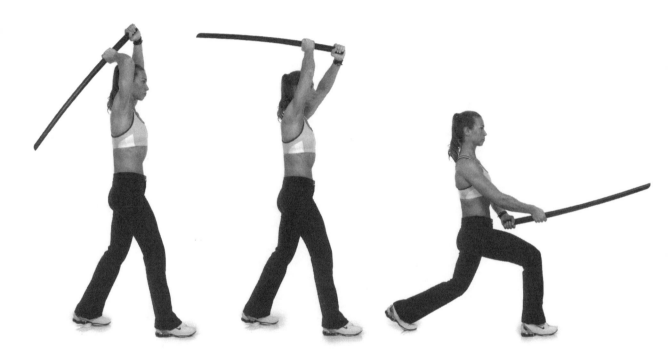

3. Twirl the sword over your right shoulder and behind your back, keeping your elbows high.

4. Strike a **Full Cut**.

Perform the exercise three to five times with your right hand on top. Then switch sides and repeat the exercise again with your left hand on top, substituting Left Step for Right Step, etc.

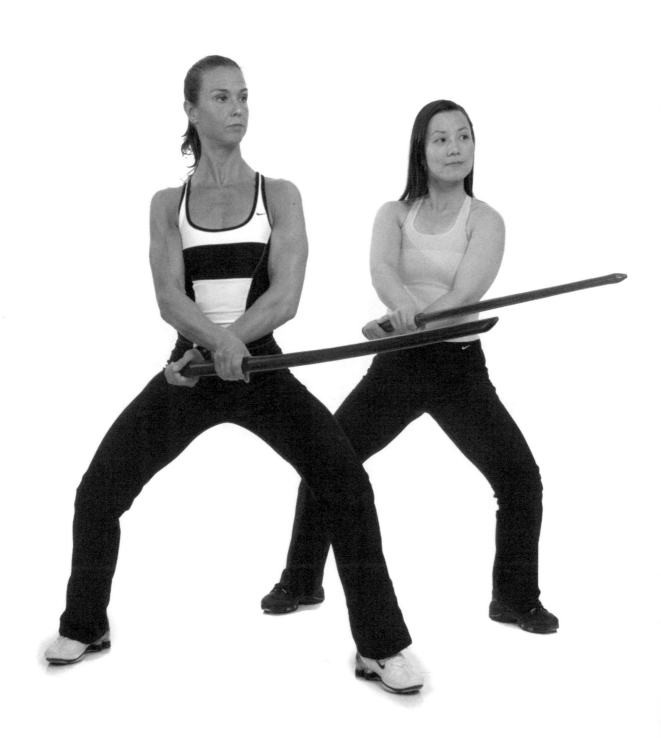

ADVANCED EXERCISES

These eight exercises cover the practice of all cuts. Remember, each exercise is performed with your right hand as the leading hand first, then with the left hand as leading hand. All exercises start and finish in the On Guard position, sword aiming at eye level as you hold the handle near your navel.

Execute each series of cuts smoothly, without pausing between them.

Advanced Exercise #1:
THE HIGH DIAGONALS

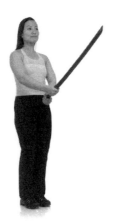

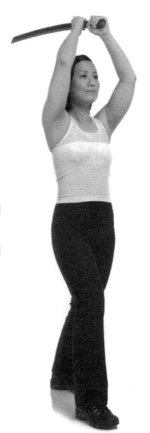

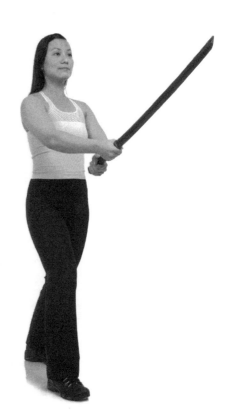

STARTING POSITION: Start with your **Feet Together** and the sword in the **On Guard** position with your right hand on top.

1. Taking a **Right Step** forward, perform a **Half Cut**.

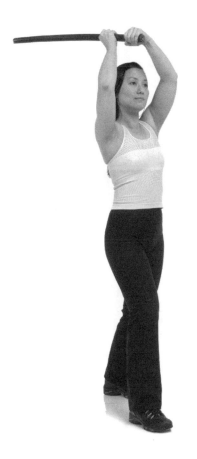
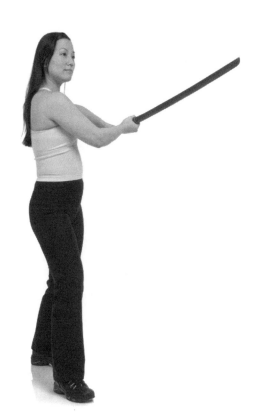

2. Perform a **Diagonal 1 High Cut** from right to left.

continued on next page →

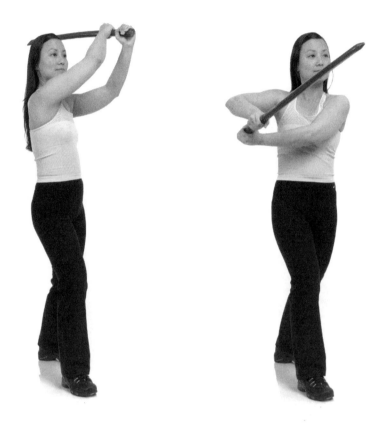

3. Perform a **Diagonal 2 High Cut** from left to right. Return to the **On Guard** position.

Repeat three to five times, then switch sides and repeat the exercise again.

Tip: Twist your shoulders and keep your weight distributed evenly between the front leg and the back leg.

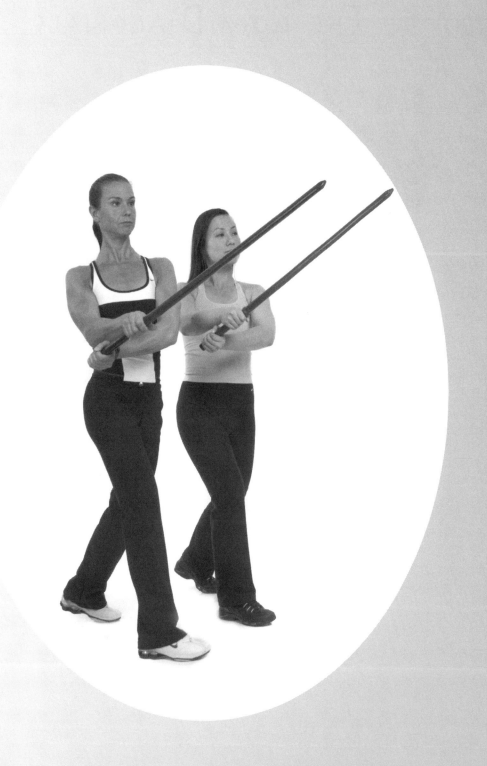

Advanced Exercise #2:
THE LOW DIAGONALS

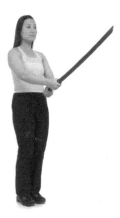

STARTING POSITION: Start with your **Feet Together** and the sword in the **On Guard** position with your right hand on top.

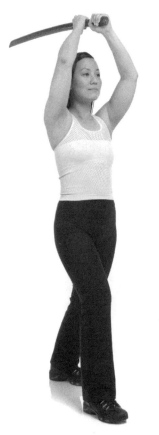

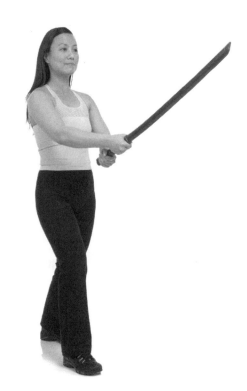

1. Taking a **Right Step** forward, perform a **Half Cut**.

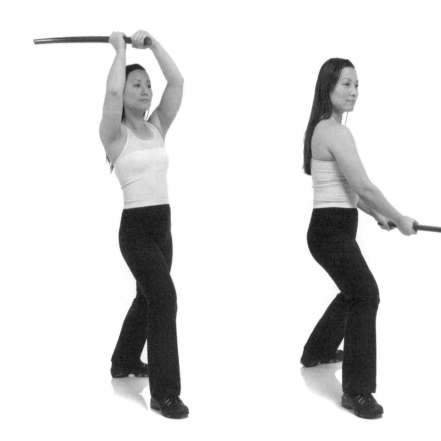

2. Perform a **Diagonal 1 Low Cut** from right to left in a **Right Lunge**.

continued on next page ⟶

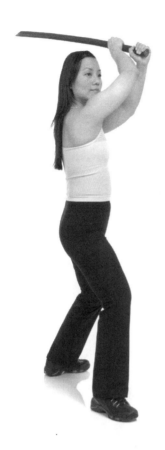 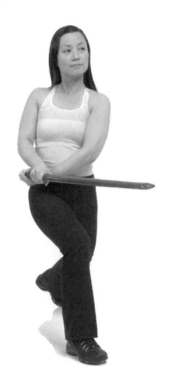

3. Still in a lunge, perform a **Diagonal 2 Low Cut** from left to right. Return to the **On Guard** position.

Repeat three to five times, then switch sides and repeat the exercise again.

Tip: Push from the right hip for the right diagonal cut (Diagonal 1) and from the left hip for the left diagonal cut (Diagonal 2), always keeping your elbows bent and close to the body.

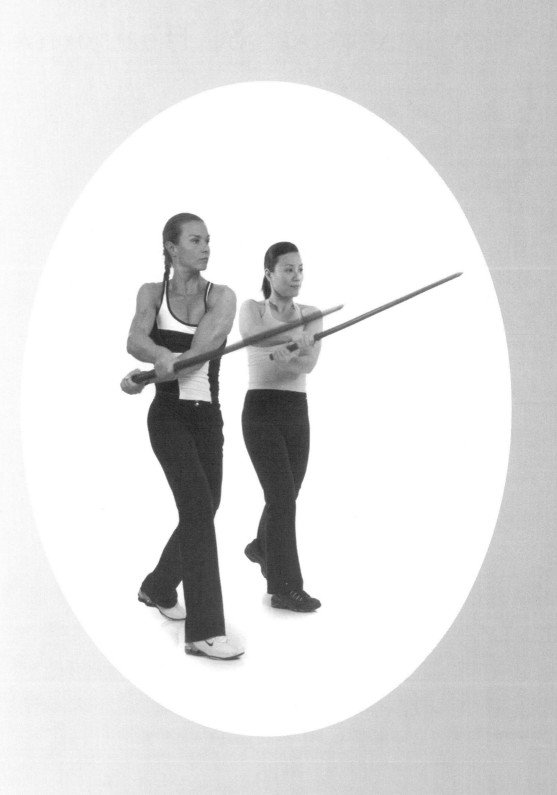

Advanced Exercise #3:
HIGH DIAGONALS & HORIZONTAL

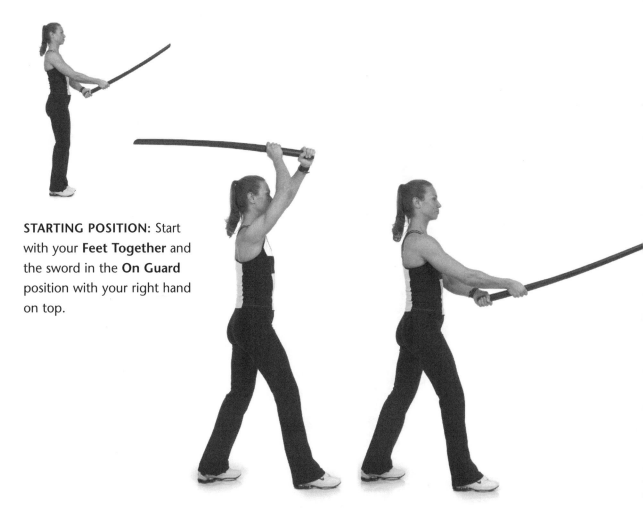

STARTING POSITION: Start with your **Feet Together** and the sword in the **On Guard** position with your right hand on top.

1. Take a **Right Step** forward and perform a **Half Cut**.

This exercise is the same as Exercise #1 with the addition of a Horizontal Cut.

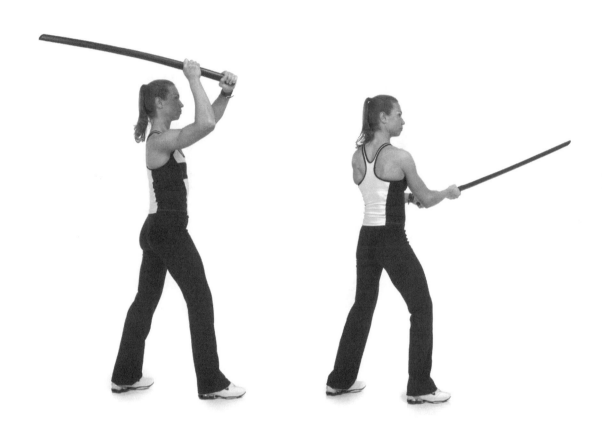

2. Perform a **Diagonal 1 High Cut** from right to left.

continued on next page →

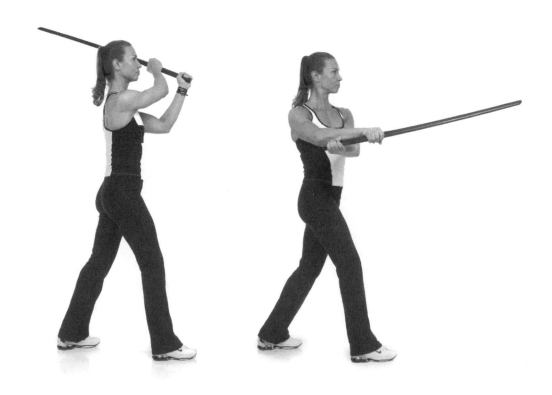

3. Perform a **Diagonal 2 High Cut** from left to right.

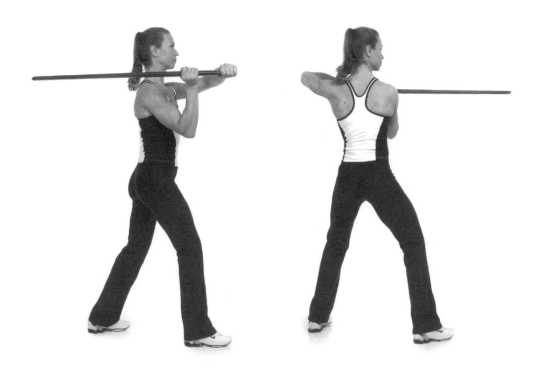

4. Perform a **Horizontal Cut** from right to left. Return to the On Guard position.

Repeat three to five times, then switch sides and repeat the exercise again.

Tip: Support the sword with your right hand and pull back from the left shoulder.

Advanced Exercise #4:

LOW HORIZONTAL

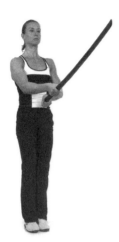

STARTING POSITION: Start with your **Feet Together** and the sword **On Guard** with your right hand on top.

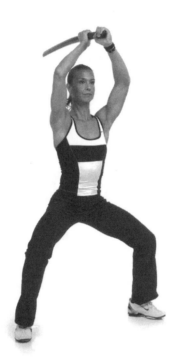

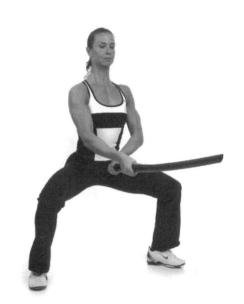

1. Sidestep **Left** into a **Squat** and perform a **Full Cut**.

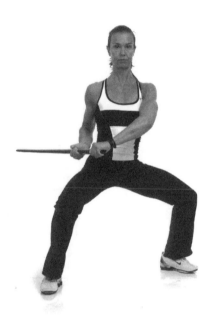 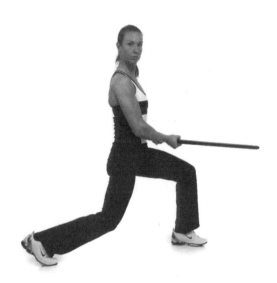

2. Perform a **Low Horizontal Cut** from right to left. Return to the On Guard position.

Repeat three to five times, then switch sides and repeat the exercise again.
Tip: Don't lean into the cut—keep your chest up.

Advanced Exercise #5:

THRUST

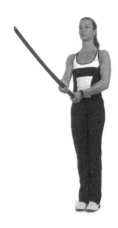

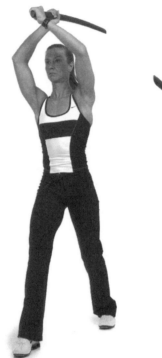

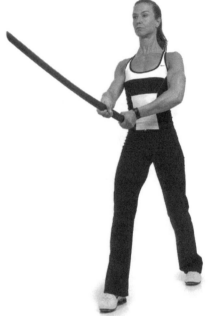

STARTING POSITION: Start with your **Feet Together** and the sword **On Guard** with your right hand on top.

1. Take a **Right Step** forward and perform a **Half Cut**.

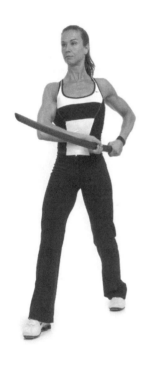

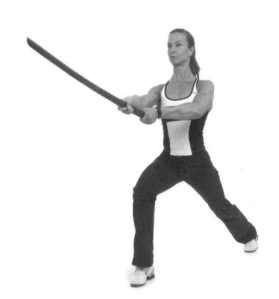

2. **Lunge Right** into a **Thrust** forward. Return to the **On Guard** position.

Repeat three to five times, then switch sides and repeat the exercise again.

Tip: Push the strike with the left leg and pull back into On Guard.

Advanced Exercise #6:

DIAGONAL 3

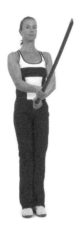

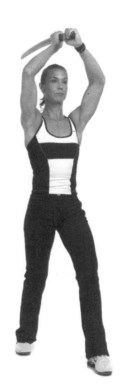

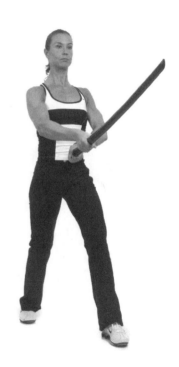

STARTING POSITION: Start with your **Feet Together** and the sword **On Guard** with your right hand on top.

1. Taking a **Left Step** forward, perform a **Half Cut**.

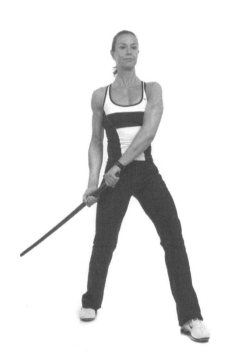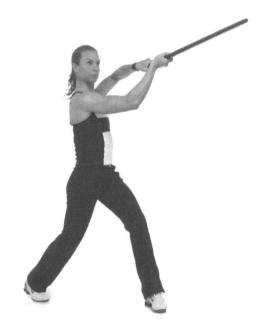

2. Step again with the left foot, bringing it more to the left side, while performing a **Diagonal 3 Cut** from right to left. Return to the **On Guard** position.

Repeat three to five times, then switch sides and repeat the exercise again.

Tip: Your left elbow should be high and your right biceps flexed as in an uppercut punch.

Advanced Exercise #7:

KENDO STRIKES

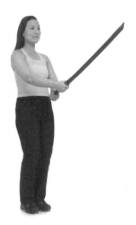

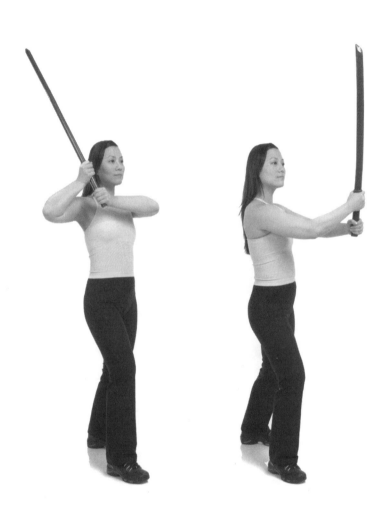

STARTING POSITION: Start with your **Feet Together** and the sword **On Guard** with your right hand on top.

1. Take a **Right Step** forward and perform four **Kendo Strikes**, shuffling forward with each strike, keeping your right foot in front.

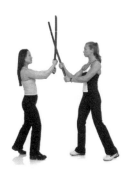

Visualize crossing swords with an imaginary opponent, like this.

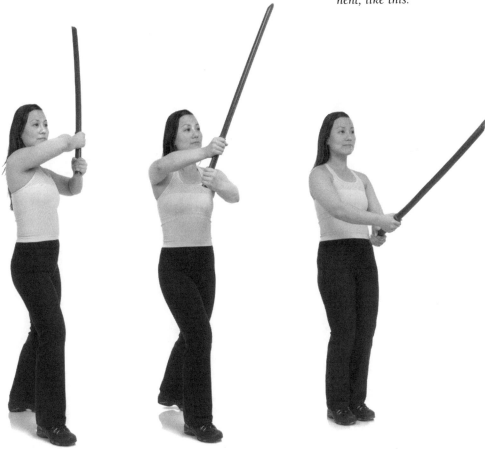

2. Bring your **Feet Together** and the sword to the **On Guard** position.

Repeat three to five times, then switch sides and repeat the exercise again.

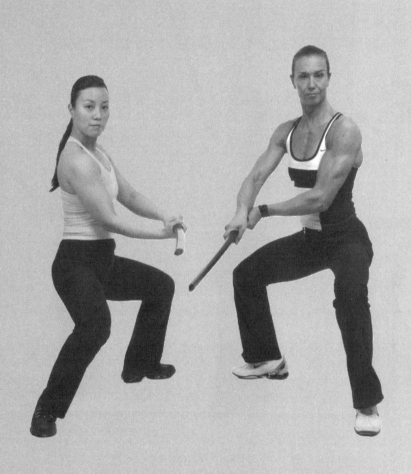

part ROUTINES three

Each routine combines several of the exercises you have practiced into a smooth sequence of choreographed movements. Practice the first routine repeatedly until you can do it easily without looking at the book. Then, proceeding at your own pace, move on to the next routine. Later you may wish to combine several routines into a longer one or experiment with creating your own routines.

ROUTINE #1: Still Water

1

Start with your **Feet Together** and the sword **On Guard**.

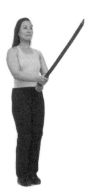

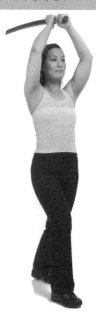

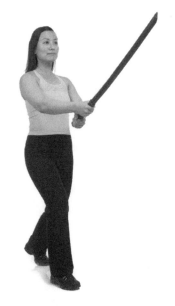

2

Take a **Right Step** forward and at the same time perform a **Half Cut**.

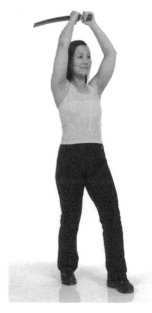

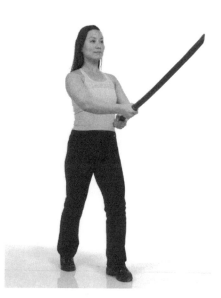

4

Bringing the sword back above your head, take a **Left Step** forward and at the same time perform a **Half Cut**.

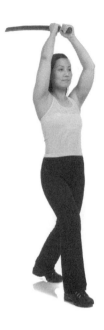
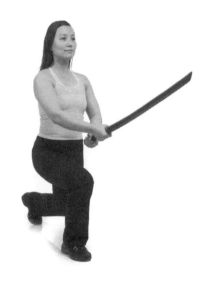

3

Bringing the sword back above your head, make a **Right Lunge** and at the same time perform a **Full Cut**.

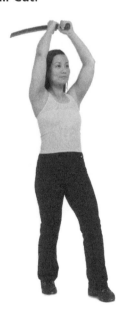
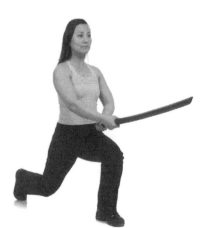

5

Bringing the sword back above your head, make a **Left Lunge** and at the same time perform a **Full Cut**.

continued on next page ⟶

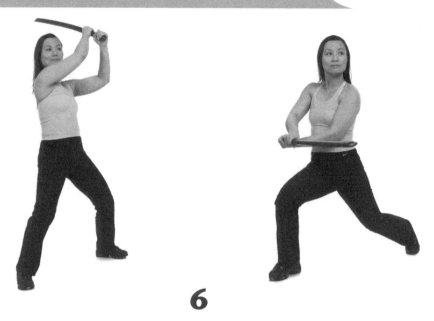

6

Moving into a **Right Squat**, perform a **Diagonal 2 Low Cut** from left to right.

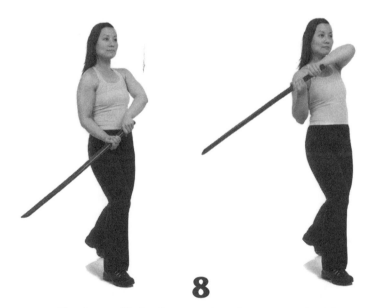

8

Rise into a **Right Step,** and perform a **Twirl with Half Cut**. Return to the **On Guard** position, **Feet Together.**

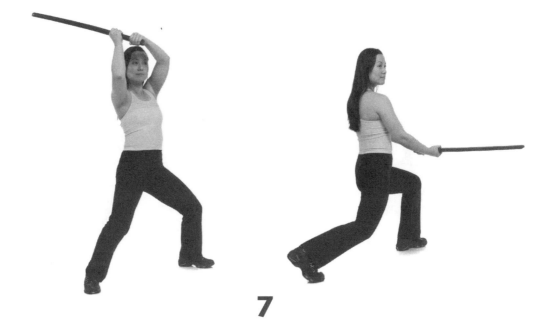

7

Moving into a **Left Squat**, perform a **Diagonal 1 Low Cut** from right to left.

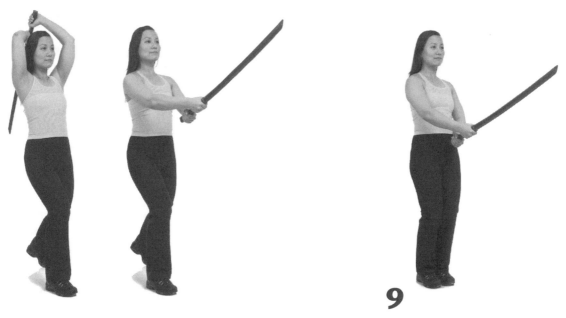

step 8 continued

9

Return to the **On Guard** position, **Feet Together**.

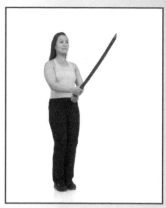

1. On Guard Feet Together

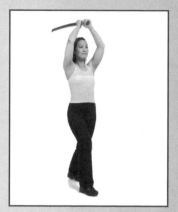

2. Right Step Half Cut

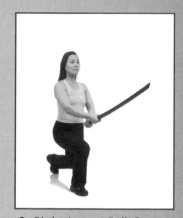

3. Right Lunge Full Cut

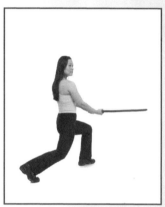

7. Left Squat Diagonal 1 Low Cut (R-L)

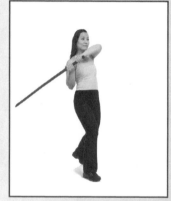

8. Right Step Twirl with Half Cut

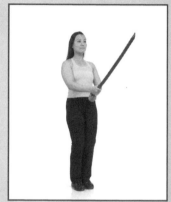

9. On Guard Feet Together

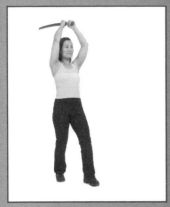

4. Left Step Half Cut

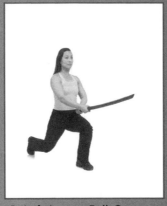

5. Left Lunge Full Cut

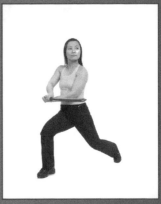

6. Right Squat Diagonal 2 Low Cut (L-R)

1

Start with your **Feet Together** and the sword **On Guard**. Execute the following cuts smoothly, without pausing.

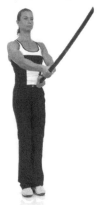

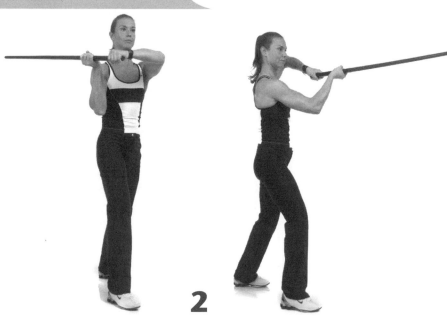

2

Take a **Right Step** forward and at the same time perform a **Horizontal Cut** from right to left.

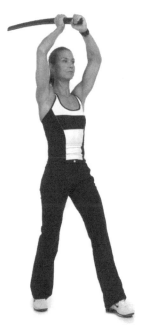

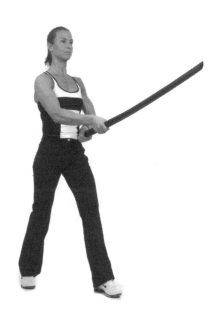

4

With your left foot still forward, perform another **Half Cut**.

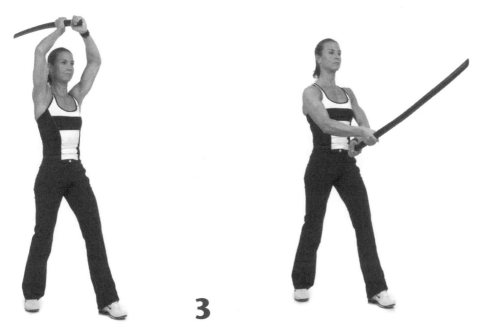

3

Take a **Left Step** forward and perform a **Half Cut**.

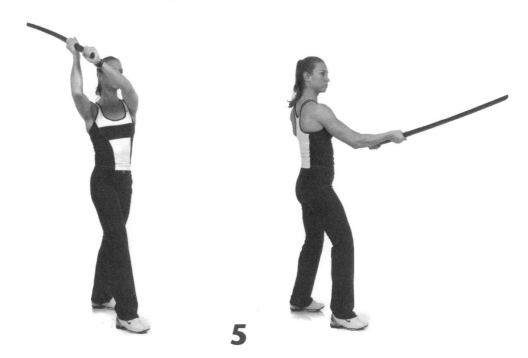

5

Take a **Right Step** forward and perform a **Diagonal
1 High Cut** from right to left.

continued on next page ⟶

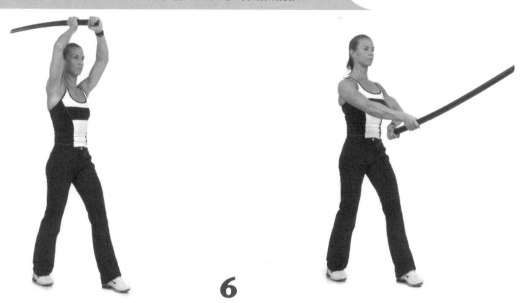

6

Take a **Left Step** forward and perform a **Half Cut**.

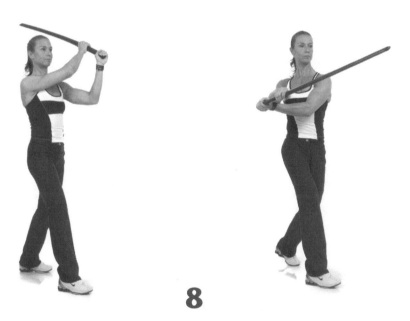

8

Take a **Right Step** forward and perform a **Diagonal 2 High Cut** from left to right.

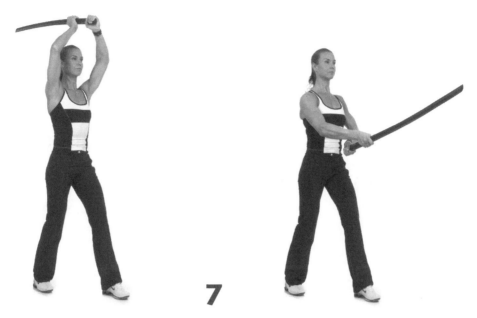

7

With your left foot still forward, perform another **Half Cut**.

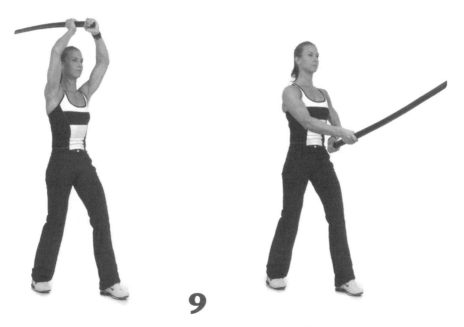

9

Take a **Left Step** forward and perform a **Half Cut**.

continued on next page →

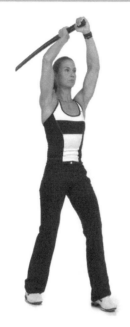

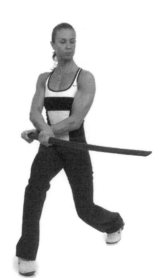

10

With your left foot still forward, perform another
Half Cut.

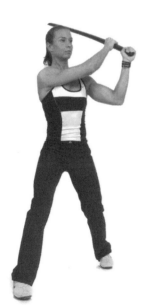

12

Still in a **Right Squat**, perform a **Diagonal 2 Low
Cut** from left to right.

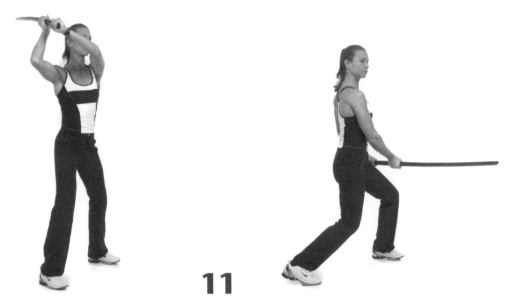

11

Sidestep **Right** into a **Squat** and perform a **Diagonal 1 Low Cut** from right to left.

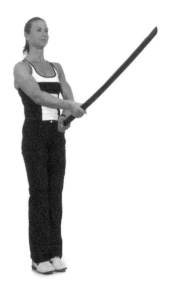

13

Return to the **On Guard** position, **Feet Together**.

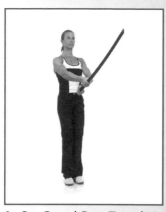

1. On Guard Feet Together

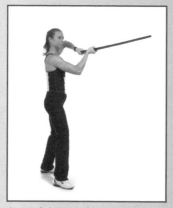

2. Right Step Horizontal Cut (R-L)

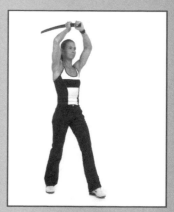

3. Left Step Half Cut

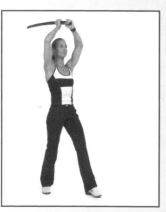

7. Half Cut

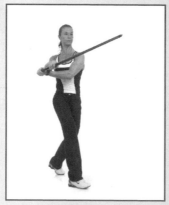

8. Right Step Diagonal 2 High Cut (L-R)

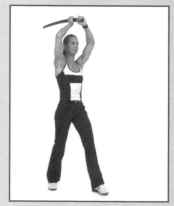

9. Left Step Half Cut

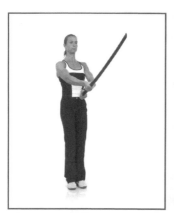

13. On Guard Feet Together

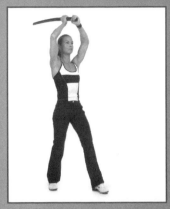

4. Half Cut

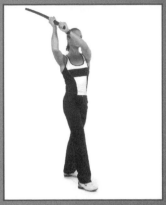

5. Right Step Diagonal 1
   High Cut (R-L)

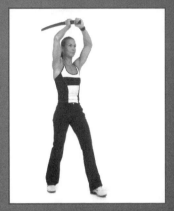

6. Left Step Half Cut

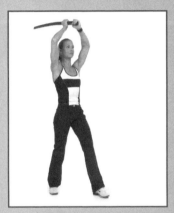

10. Half Cut

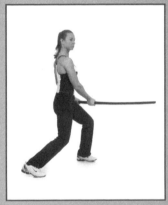

11. Right Squat Diagonal 1
    Low Cut (R-L)

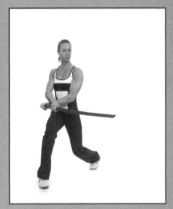

12. Right Squat Diagonal 2
    Low Cut (L-R)

1

Start with your **Feet Together** and the sword **On Guard**. Execute the following cuts smoothly, without pausing. The first three cuts should be performed in fast sequence, without a break.

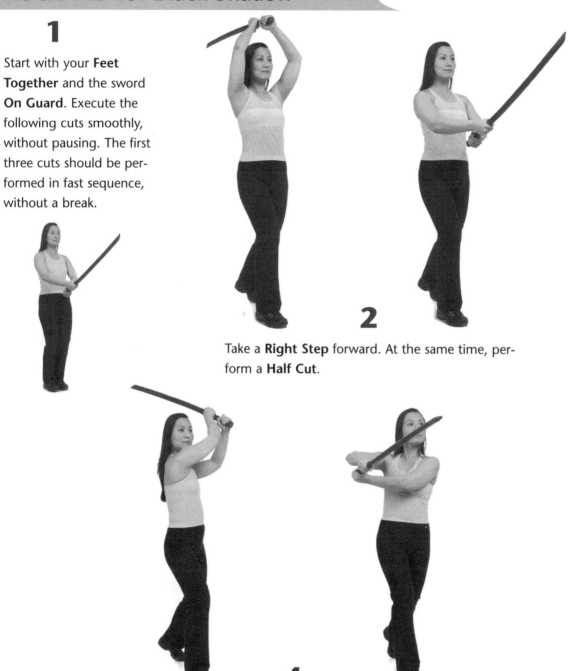

2

Take a **Right Step** forward. At the same time, perform a **Half Cut**.

4

Perform a **Diagonal 2 High Cut** from left to right.

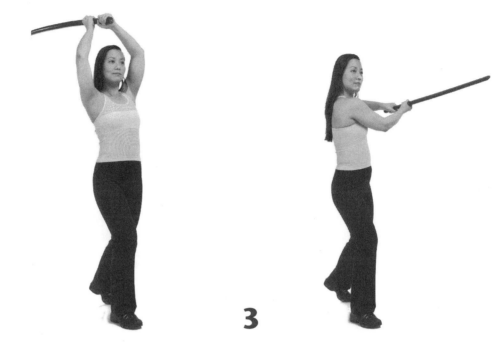

3

Perform a **Diagonal 1 High Cut** from right to left.

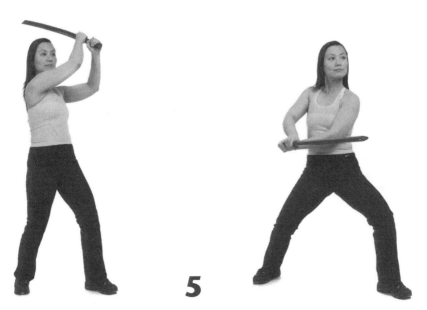

5

Take a **Left Step** forward. At the same time, perform a **Diagonal 2 Low Cut** from left to right, going into a **Left Lunge**.

continued on next page ⟶

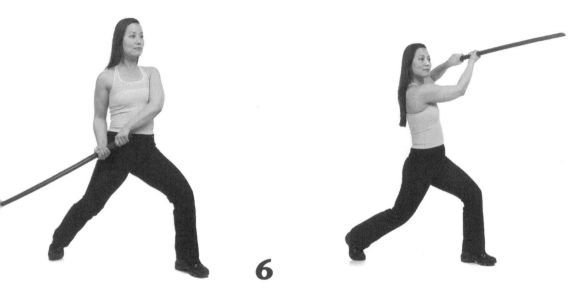

6

Perform a **Diagonal 3 Cut** from right to left.

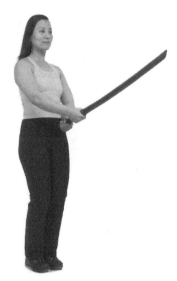

8

Return to the **On Guard** position, **Feet Together**.

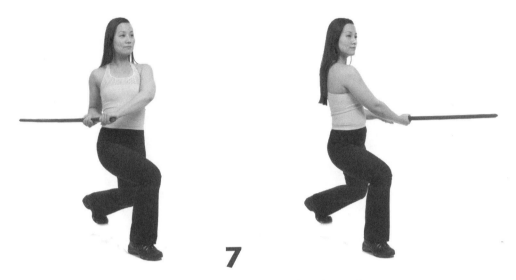

7

Move into a **Right Lunge** while performing a **Low Horizontal Cut** from left to right.

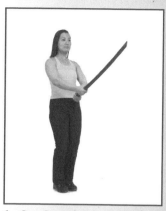

1. On Guard Feet Together

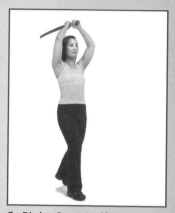

2. Right Step Half Cut

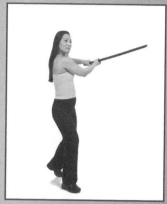

3. Diagonal 1 High Cut (R-L)

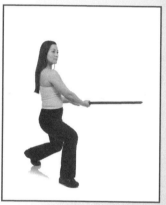

7. Right Lunge Low Horizontal Cut (L-R)

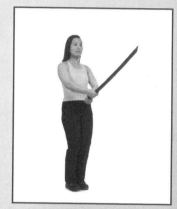

8. On Guard Feet Together

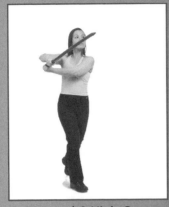

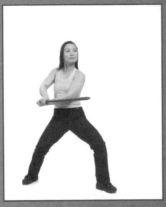

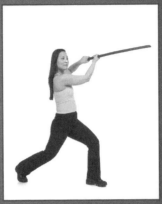

4. Diagonal 2 High Cut
   (L-R)

5. Left Step Diagonal 2
   Low Cut (L-R) Lunge

6. Diagonal 3 Cut (R-L)

ROUTINE #4: Panther

1

Start with your **Feet Together** and the sword **On Guard**. Execute the following cuts smoothly, without pausing.

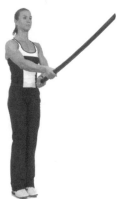

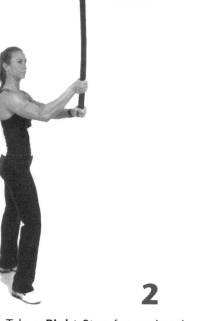

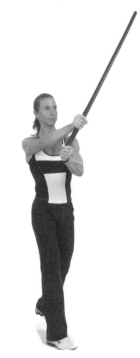

2

Take a **Right Step** forward and make four **Kendo Strikes**, shuffling forward with each strike, keeping your right foot forward.

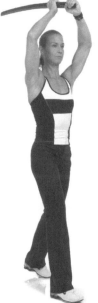

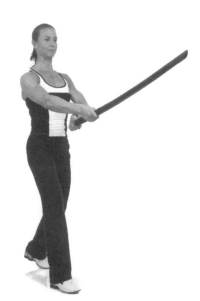

3

Perform a **Half Cut**.

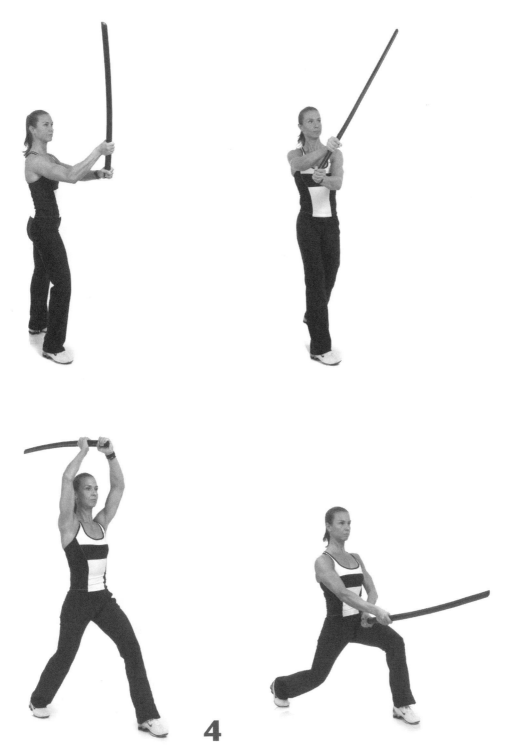

4

Step into a **Left Lunge** and perform a **Full Cut**.

continued on next page ⟶

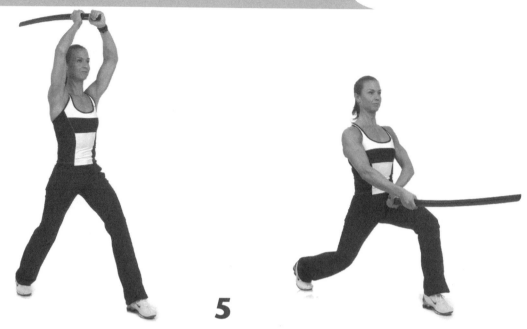

5

Still in a lunge, perform another **Full Cut**.

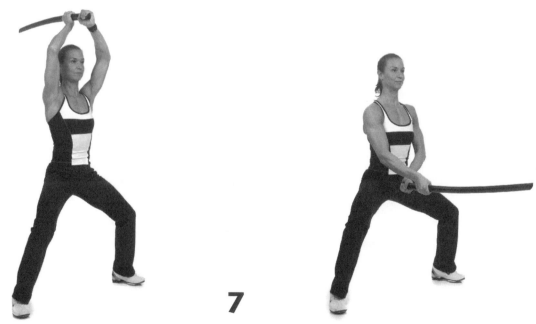

7

Sidestep **Left** into a **Squat** and perform another **Full Cut**.

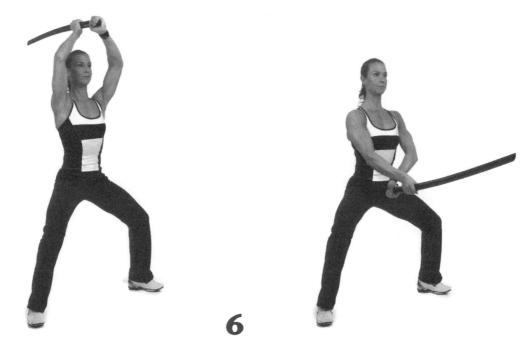

6

Sidestep **Right** into a **Squat** and at the same time perform another **Full Cut**.

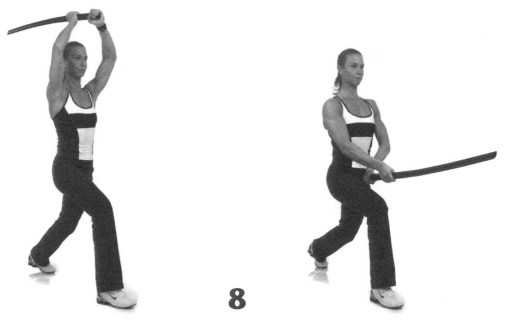

8

Move into a **Right Lunge** while performing a **Full Cut**.

continued on next page ➞

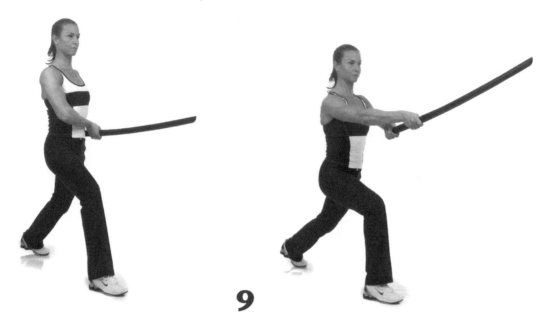

9

Still in a lunge, perform a **Thrust**.

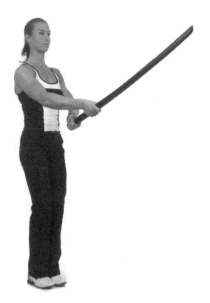

10

Return to the **On Guard** position, **Feet Together.**

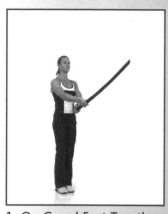

1. On Guard Feet Together

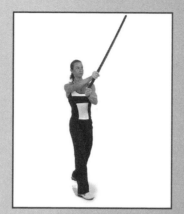

2. Four Kendo Strikes

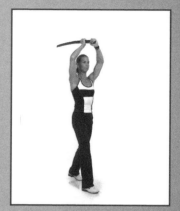

3. Half Cut

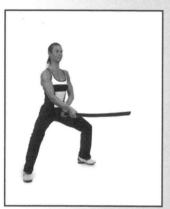

7. Left Squat Full Cut

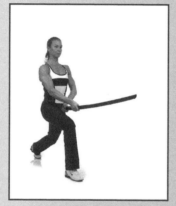

8. Right Lunge Full Cut

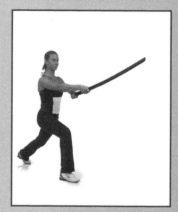

9. Thrust

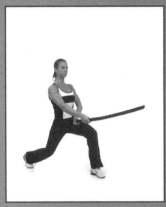 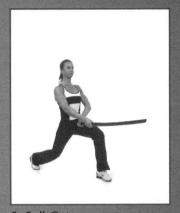 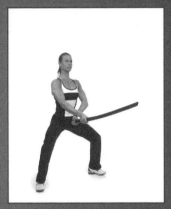

4. Left Lunge Full Cut

5. Full Cut

6. Right Squat Full Cut

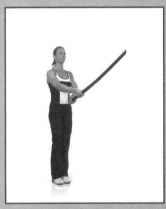

10. On Guard Feet
    Together

1

Start with your **Feet Together** and the sword **On Guard**. Execute the following cuts smoothly, without pausing.

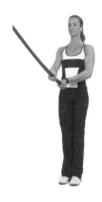

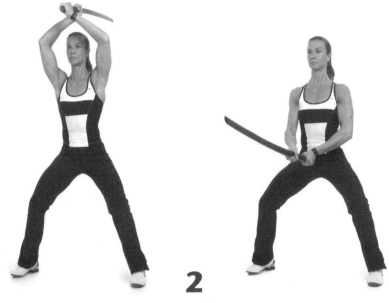

2

Sidestep **Right** into a **Squat** and perform a **Full Cut**.

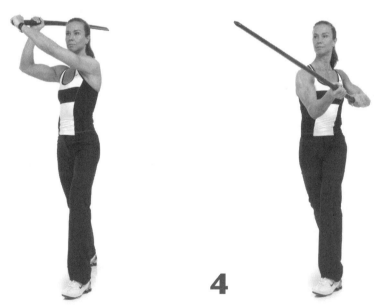

4

Take a **Left Step** forward while performing a **Diagonal 1 High Cut** from right to left.

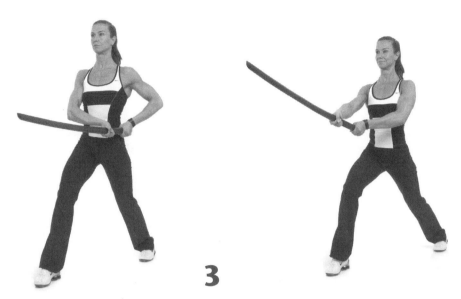

3

Move into a **Right Lunge** while performing a **Thrust**.

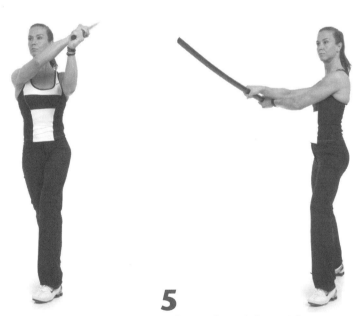

5

Perform a **Diagonal 2 High Cut** from left to right.

continued on next page →

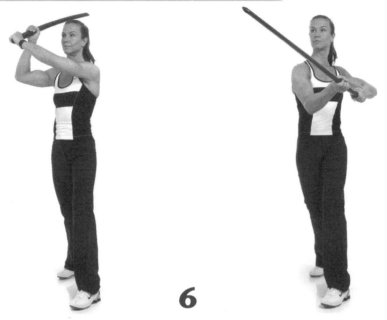

6

Repeat the **Diagonal 1 High Cut** from right to left.

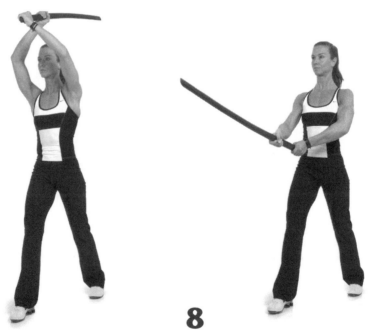

8

Take a **Right Step** forward while performing a **Half Cut**.

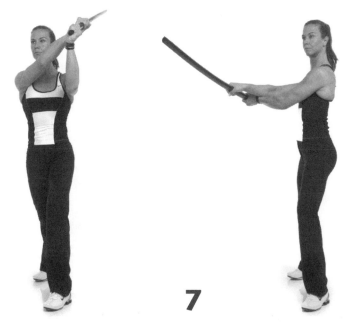

7

Repeat the **Diagonal 2 High Cut** from left to right.

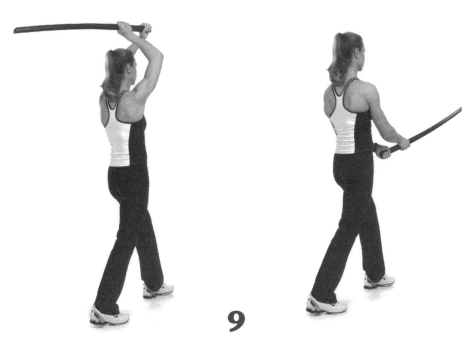

9

Pivot to the rear, with your left foot forward, and perform a **Half Cut**.

continued on next page ⟶

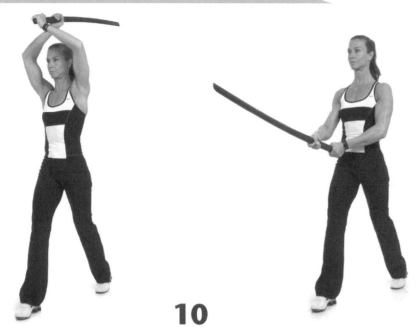

10

Pivot to the front, with your right foot forward, and perform a **Half Cut**.

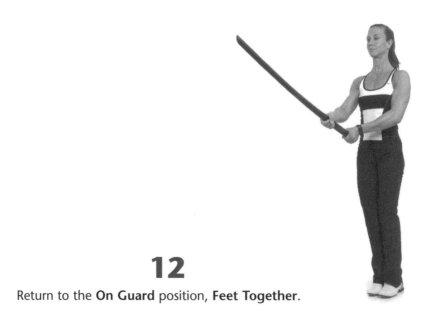

12

Return to the **On Guard** position, **Feet Together**.

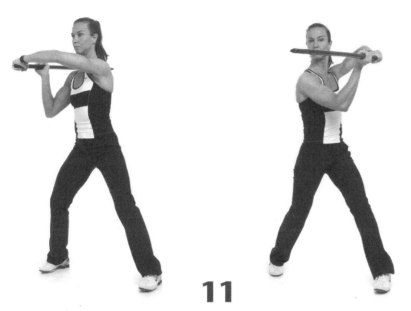

11

Sidestep **Left** into a **Squat** and perform a **Horizontal Cut**.

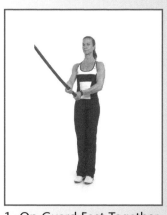

1. On Guard Feet Together

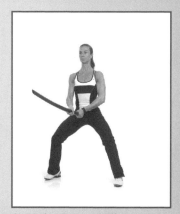

2. Right Squat Full Cut

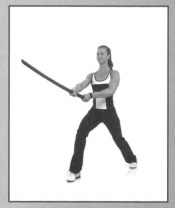

3. Right Lunge Thrust

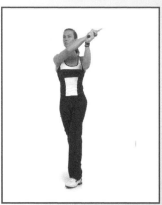

7. Diagonal 2 High Cut
   (L-R)

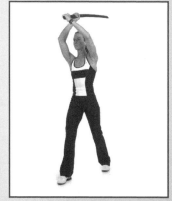

8. Right Step Half Cut

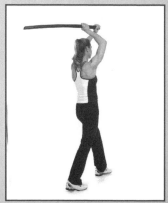

9. Pivot Half Cut

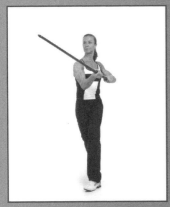

4. Left Step Diagonal 1
   High Cut (R-L)

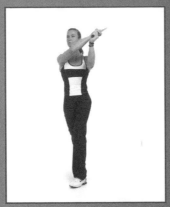

5. Diagonal 2 High Cut
   (L-R)

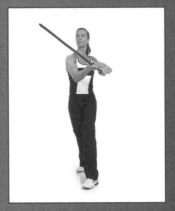

6. Diagonal 1 High Cut
   (R-L)

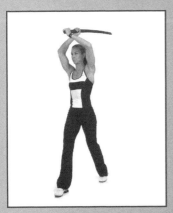

10. Pivot Half Cut

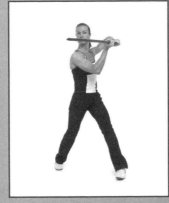

11. Left Squat Horizontal
    Cut

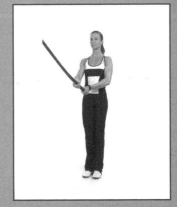

12. On Guard Feet
    Together

ROUTINE #6: Samurai

1

Start with your **Feet Together** and the sword **On Guard**. Execute the following cuts smoothly, without pausing.

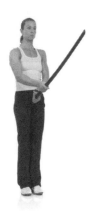

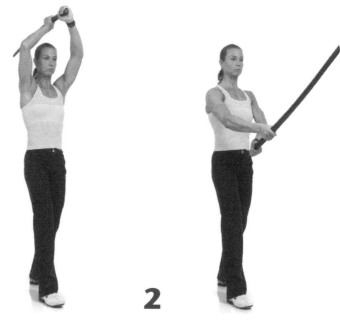

2

Take a **Right Step** forward. At the same time perform a **Half Cut**.

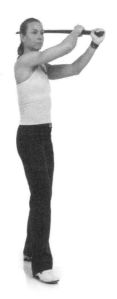

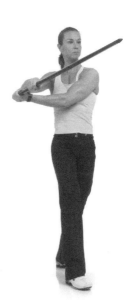

4

Perform a **Diagonal 2 High Cut** from left to right.

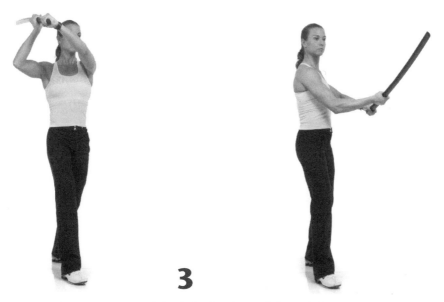

3

Perform a **Diagonal 1 High Cut** from right to left.

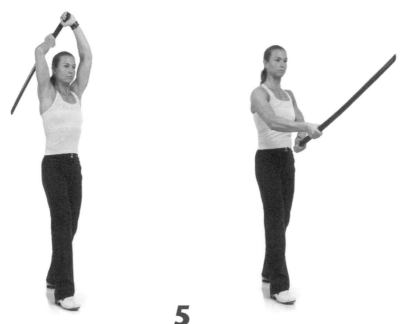

5

Perform a **Twirl with a Half Cut**.

continued on next page →

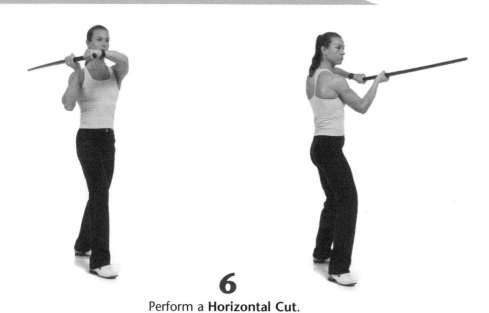

6

Perform a **Horizontal Cut**.

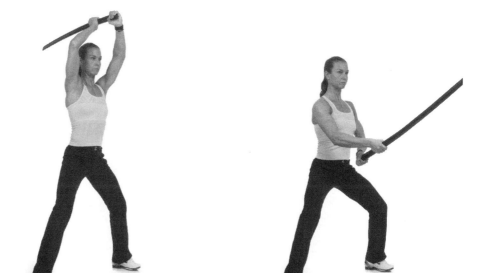

8

Move into a **Squat** and perform a **Half Cut**.

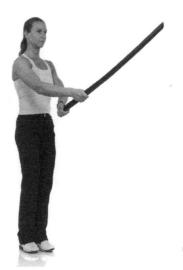

7

Return to the **On Guard** position with your **Feet Together**.

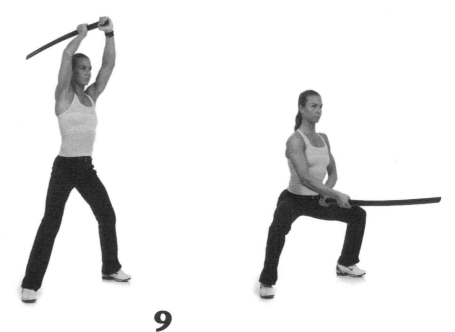

9

Still in a **Squat**, perform a **Full Cut**.

continued on next page →

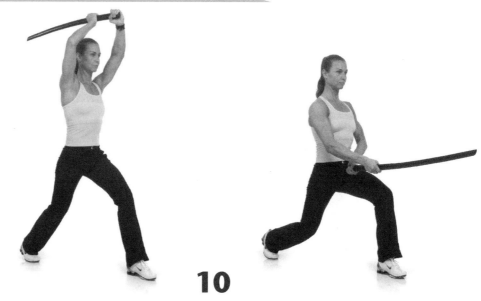

10

Rotate your feet into a **Left Lunge** while performing a **Full Cut**.

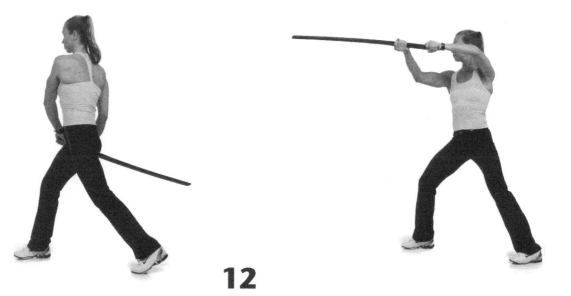

12

Perform a **Diagonal 3 Cut** from right to left.

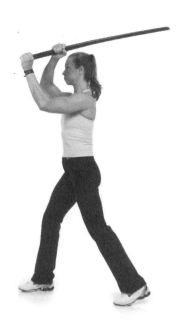 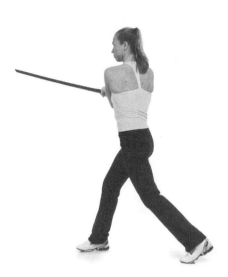

11

Pivot to the back, with your right foot forward, then perform a **Diagonal 2 High Cut** from left to right.

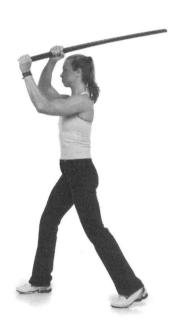 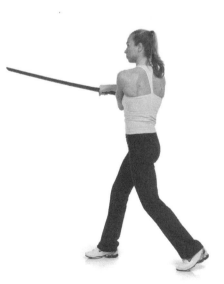

13

Perform a **Diagonal 2 High Cut** from left to right.

continued on next page →

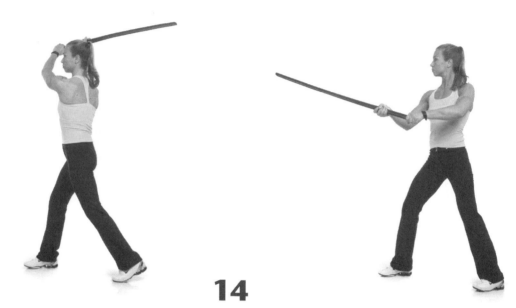

14

Perform a **Diagonal 1 High Cut** from right to left.

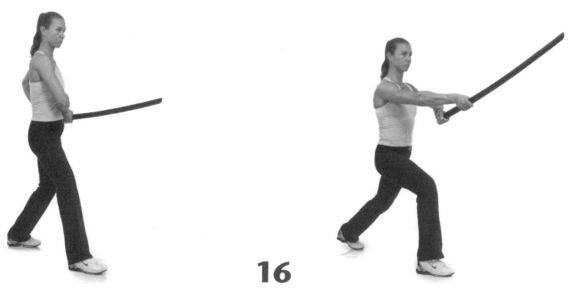

16

Make a **Right Lunge** while performing a **Thrust**.

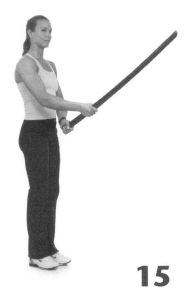

15

Pivot and return to the **On Guard** position with your **Feet Together**.

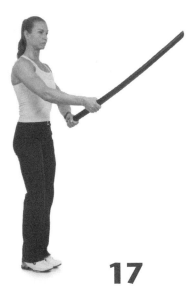

17

Return to the **On Guard** position with your **Feet Together**.

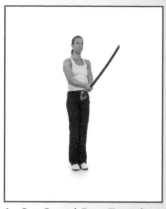

1. On Guard Feet Together

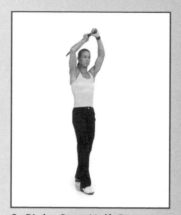

2. Right Step Half Cut

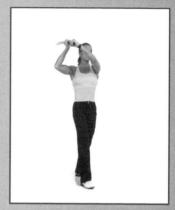

3. Diagonal 1 High Cut (R-L)

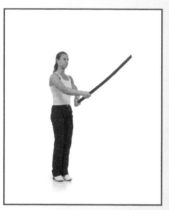

7. On Guard Feet Together

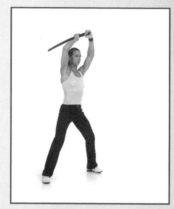

8. Squat Half Cut

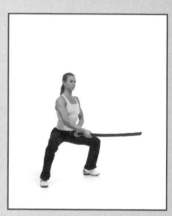

9. Full Cut

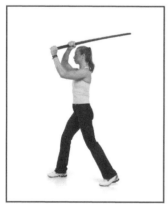

13. Diagonal 2 High Cut (L-R)

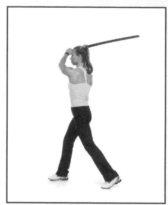

14. Diagonal 1 High Cut (R-L)

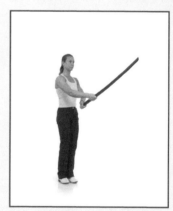

15. Pivot On Guard Feet Together

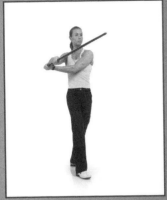

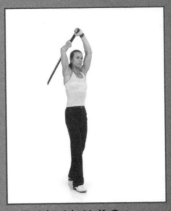

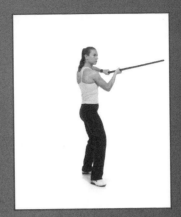

4. Diagonal 2 High Cut (L-R)

5. Twirl with Half Cut

6. Horizontal Cut

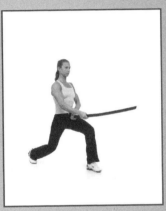

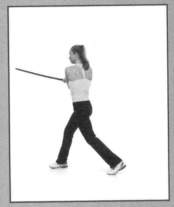

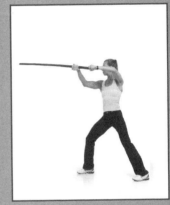

10. Left Lunge Full Cut

11. Pivot Diagonal 2 High Cut (L-R)

12. Diagonal 3 Cut (R-L)

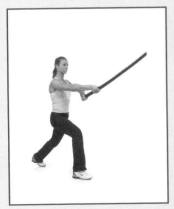

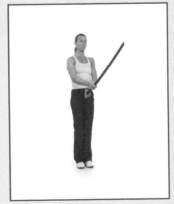

16. Right Lunge Thrust

17. On Guard Feet Together

ROUTINE #7: Blue Snow

1

Start with your **Feet Together** and the sword **On Guard**. Execute the following cuts smoothly, without pausing.

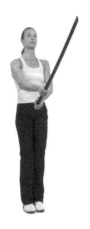

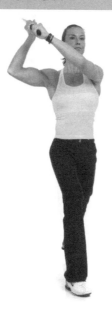

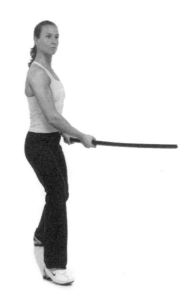

2

Step back with your left foot, bringing yourself into a **Right Stance,** and perform a **Diagonal 1 Low Cut** from right to left.

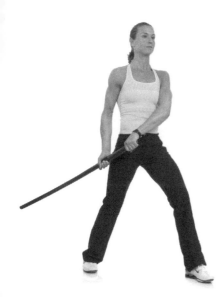

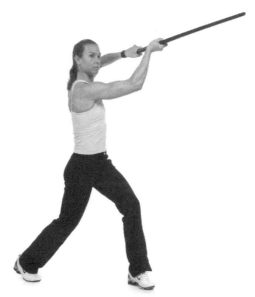

4

Take a **Left Step** forward while performing a **Diagonal 3 Cut** from right to left.

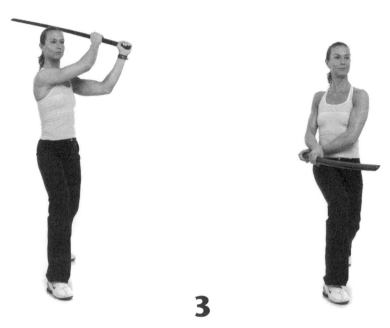

3

Perform a **Diagonal 2 Low Cut** from left to right.

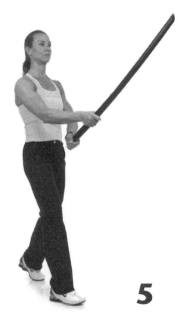

5

Step back again with your left foot into a **Right Stance** while bringing the sword to the **On Guard** position.

continued on next page →

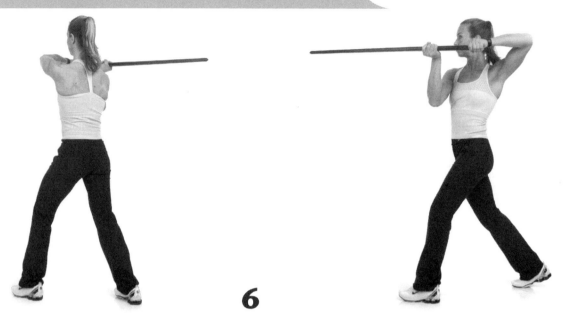

6

Pivot to the rear and perform a **Horizontal Cut**.

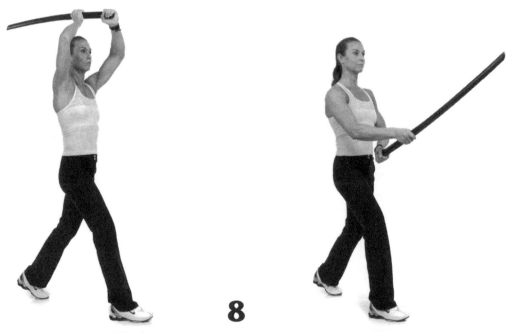

8

Pivot to the front and perform a **Half Cut**.

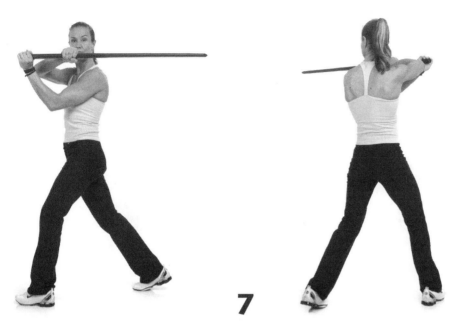

7

Perform a **Reversed Horizontal Cut**.

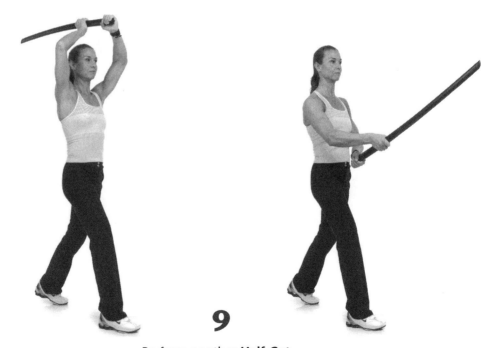

9

Perform another **Half Cut**.

continued on next page →

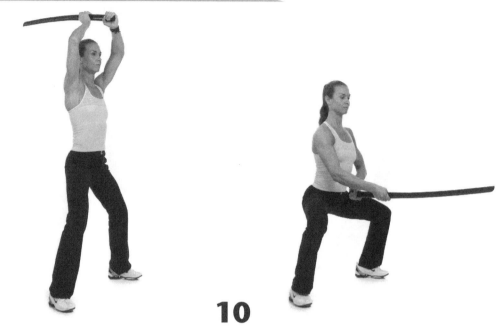

10

Sidestep **Left** into a **Squat**, and perform a **Full Cut**.

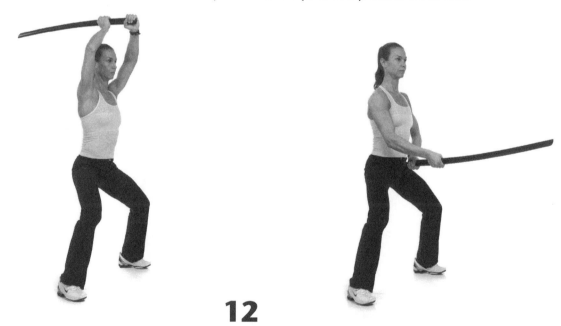

12

Hop up and sidestep **Left** into a **Squat** again for
another **Full Cut**.

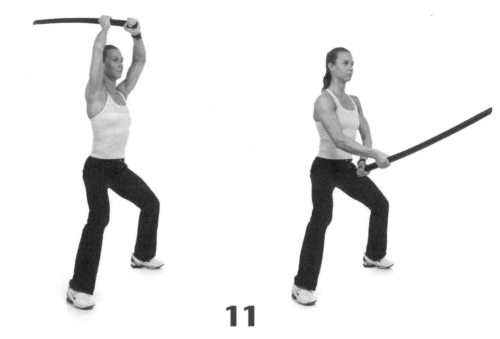

11

Hop up and sidestep **Right** into a **Squat** and perform another **Full Cut**.

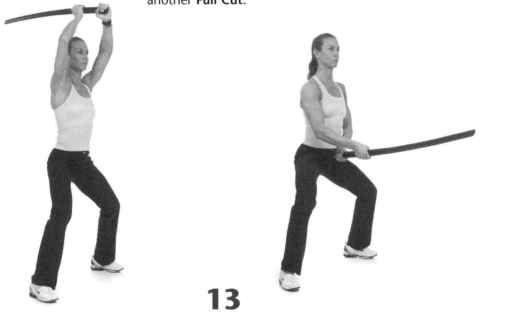

13

Hop up and sidestep **Right** into a **Squat** again for another **Full Cut**.

continued on next page ⟶

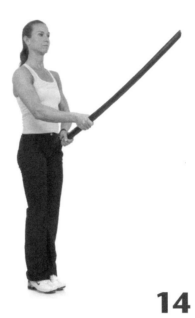

14

Stand up into the **On Guard** position with your **Feet Together**.

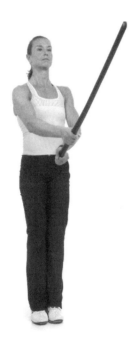

16

Return to the **On Guard** position with your **Feet Together**.

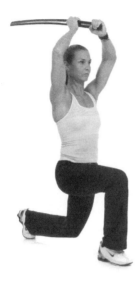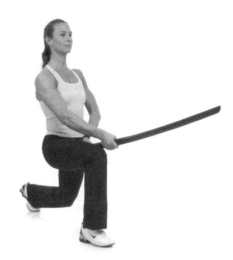

15

Step back with your left leg into a low **Right Lunge** position, with the left knee almost on the floor, and perform a very slow, deliberate **Full Cut**.

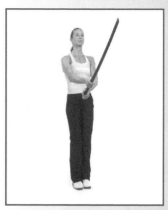

1. Feet Together On Guard

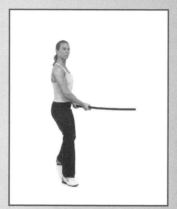

2. Step Back Right Stance Diagonal 1 Low Cut (R-L)

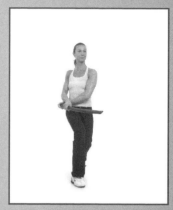

3. Diagonal 2 Low Cut (L-R)

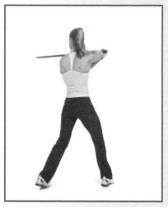

7. Reversed Horizontal Cut

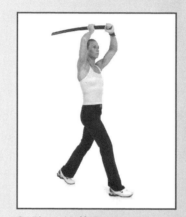

8. Pivot Half Cut

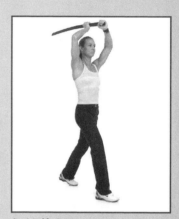

9. Half Cut

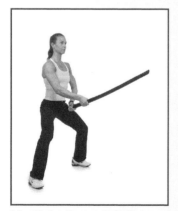

13. Right Squat Full Cut

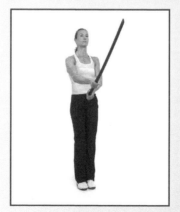

14. On Guard Feet Together

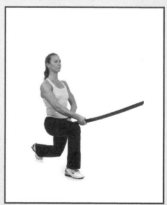

15. Step Back Right Lunge Full Cut

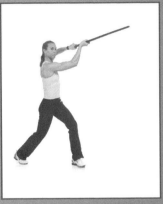

4. Left Step Diagonal 3 Cut
   (R-L)

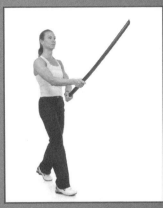

5. Step Back Right Stance
   On Guard

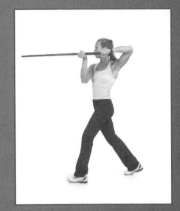

6. Pivot Horizontal Cut

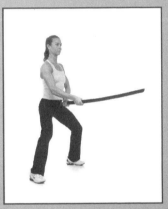

10. Left Squat Full Cut

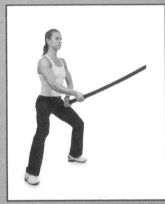

11. Right Squat Full Cut

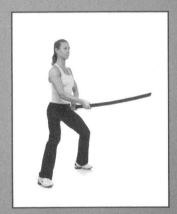

12. Left Squat Full Cut

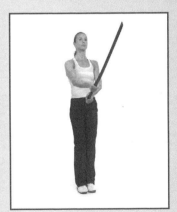

16. On Guard Feet
    Together

ABOUT THE AUTHOR

A gifted teacher with innovative ideas, **Ilaria Montagnani** is an unstoppable force in fitness. Since 1987 when Ilaria touched down in New York City from her native Italy, she has carved out a new niche in the fitness world. Recently selected as a Nike Fitness Athlete and named by *New York Magazine* as one of the leading fitness "gurus" in the city, Ilaria has transformed the practice of martial arts and become one of the most well-respected and sought after professionals in the fitness industry. With a black belt in Shorinjiru Karate and over twelve years of training in kickboxing and Samurai sword fighting, Ilaria intertwines high intensity training with the Zen of martial arts.

Ilaria is the President of Powerstrike, Inc., which was founded in 1995. Teachers throughout the world as well in the U.S. are skillfully trained in the Powerstrike programs. Ilaria has made television appearances on ABC's "Good Morning America," CBS and ABC "Evening News," "Inside Edition," "The Rosie O'Donnell Show," "NBC Weekend" and "E! Entertainment," to name a few. Recently, *The New York Post* compared Montagnani to Lara Croft: "Meet the Lara Croft of Manhattan with her slicked back-hair and six-pack abs."

ABOUT THE PHOTOGRAPHER AND MODEL

Bill Morris is a fashion and beauty photographer based in New York City. After assisting some of NY's top photographers and breaking some ground in the field himself, Bill decided to open his own studio in Soho. Since doing so he has shot over 200 national and international magazine covers. Some of Bill's clients past and present include: ABC television, Calvin Klein, Christian Dior, Clairol, and Guinness Beer.

Irene Wong is a Director of Programming at the Food Network, specializing in discovering on-air talent and developing new series. She earned a black belt in Tae Kwon Do and continues to train her mind and body through Japanese swordfighting.